FAITHFUL BEGINNINGS

Faithful Beginnings

A Doula's Guide To Eliminating Fear And Birthing With Confidence

Emmy Robbin

Published by Game Changer Publishing

Paperback **ISBN**: 978-1-965653-64-7

Hardcover **ISBN**: 978-1-965653-65-4

Digital **ISBN**: 978-1-965653-66-1

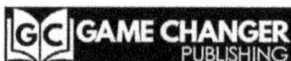
www.GameChangerPublishing.com

DEDICATION

I dedicate this book to my incredible family—my loving and supportive husband and my beautiful children, who have transformed me in so many ways. I also want to dedicate this book to all the mothers and fathers who have trusted me to be in their birth space, postpartum space, healing journey, and empowerment journey. Let's change the world by showing them how powerful we truly are when we trust God's design in us.

READ THIS FIRST

Thank you so much for purchasing my book.
Scan the QR code below for a 100% off coupon
to one of my masterminds!

Scan the QR Code:

SCAN ME

FAITHFUL BEGINNINGS
A Doula's Guide To Eliminating Fear And Birthing With Confidence

EMMY ROBBIN

CONTENTS

Introduction   xi

1. Redemption   1
2. The Physiology of Birth   7
3. Health and Wellness in Pregnancy   17
4. Intervention and Disrupting Nature's Design   23
5. Choosing Your Birth Team   31
6. The Ways Labor Begins   37
7. Breaking Down the Fears   41
8. Embracing Nature and Surrender   49
9. VBAC Is Low Risk   57
10. Faith Over Fear   63
11. Breastfeeding and Leaps   69
12. Postpartum Rest and Recovery   75
13. Birth Stories   81

Conclusion   105

INTRODUCTION

I want to preface that I am not a doctor. I am a believer in Christ and God. As a doula, I have witnessed almost every kind of birth, from hospital birth to unassisted home birth. My opinion on undisturbed physiological birth and beyond is a combination of my education in anatomy and physiology, childbirth education, being a support to so many births in the past 5 years, and how I feel that God has led me with His message. I believe that when a woman experiences birth the way He designed, there is no other empowering transformation like it.

Home birth is such a beautiful experience that all women who desire it should be free and able to choose it. I love the fact that women have access to midwifery services at home in this country (in most states... not all) so that they can experience this life-changing journey. My wish with this book is that it will teach you how the physiological process of birth works, what variations can occur, and, from there, how to advocate for yourself versus seeking outside validation or advice without informed consent or alternatives. You hold the power to your autonomy, and I hope this book inspires you to maintain that throughout your birth and postpartum journey into parenthood.

Birth is a sacred process intricately designed by God. It is a powerful, natural experience that, when undisturbed, unfolds as He intended—beautifully and perfectly. However, in our modern world, this truth has been overshadowed by fear, interventions, and a lack of faith in the body's divine design. My own journey to understanding the power of undisturbed physiological birth began after my first birth experience, which ended in a C-section, an event that shook my trust in my body. It wasn't until the "redemption birth" of my second daughter at home at the age of 41 that I *fully* realized how our bodies *are* capable of incredible, transformative birth experiences.

This book is for the woman (and her partner) who doubts, who has experienced birth trauma, or who simply wants to understand how God created birth to be. It's a guide to empowering yourself through knowledge, faith, and preparation to reclaim birth as the natural, instinctual process it is: mammalian birth. Together, we'll explore not only the mechanics of physiological birth but also the deep spiritual and emotional aspects that shape it. I hope that by the end, you'll be inspired to trust the body God gave you and feel confident in your ability to birth naturally and powerfully.

CHAPTER ONE
REDEMPTION

"Perhaps this is the moment for which you were created."
—Esther 4:14

The fact that an entire chapter on redemptive birth is necessary saddens me deeply, both as a mother and a doula. Many of the women I support, including myself, have sought redemption in birth—often looking back and wishing they could have experienced that bliss the first time around. As a doula, my mission is to empower and educate as many people as possible—women and their partners—about the beauty and wisdom of undisturbed physiological birth. From this foundation of knowledge, they can make informed decisions about any interventions offered, weighing risks and benefits in a way that allows them to retain control and empowerment.

Transformative, powerful, beautiful, magical, and life-changing—birth has the potential to be all of these things and more. To achieve this, education and the dissolution of fear are crucial. My hope is that by learning about physiological birth, more women can experience their births as truly empowering events.

From the time we are young girls, we are conditioned to seek external validation to understand our bodies. Our education fails us by not teaching us the intricate processes of menstruation, conception, birth, or breastfeeding. Most of us receive nothing more than a brief, often inadequate, sex education class. My own experience was a 25-minute lecture that included a horrifying video of a woman screaming while giving birth. It left me at age 15 to declare, "I'm never doing that."

We aren't taught about the menstrual cycle—the four phases we experience and how they affect us physically and emotionally —or how to properly care for ourselves during these times. We certainly aren't taught about the physiological marvel that is conception, how intricately and perfectly God designed this process. I believe this lack of knowledge, among other things, contributes to the infertility crisis we see today.

Boys are taught that menstruation is gross, while girls are taught to feel shame about their natural cycles. The importance of nutrition, stress management, hydration, movement, and mindfulness is often absent from our upbringing. We are not taught about the critical role of oxytocin, not only in birth but in bonding, breastfeeding, and even everyday life. Most women have never even seen another woman breastfeed before they have their first baby, making the experience foreign and overwhelming.

This is why I decided to write this book. My name is Emmy Robbin. I'm a doula, birth keeper, childbirth educator, lactation counselor, birth trauma healing coach, wife, podcast host, actress, and mother to two beautiful daughters. My limited exposure to childbirth growing up came through my family—my mother's birth stories, in particular. However, these stories were not empowering. They were laced with trauma and fear. My mother's experience with my brother involved being "knocked out," so she barely remembers his birth. With my sister, my mother recalled how she "went down the wrong way and broke my tailbone." Sadly, I never heard my own birth story. My mother passed away after a long battle with breast cancer when I was 25.

As a child and teenager, witnessing my mother's illness took a heavy toll on my nervous system, contributing to issues with my menstrual cycle and eventually leading to a diagnosis of poly-cystic ovary syndrome (PCOS) and a rare blood disorder called Von-Willebrand's disease. At nine years old, I also had my appendix removed due to a condition called lymph node hyper-plasia. My story exemplifies the deep connection between our mental, emotional, and physical health, which becomes especially relevant during conception, pregnancy, birth, and beyond.

Being diagnosed with PCOS at a young age put me under the constant supervision of gynecologists. Birth control pills were prescribed to manage my symptoms, and every doctor's visit seemed to bring more dire warnings about my fertility. I was told that without intervention, I would likely struggle to conceive. Never was the role of nutrition or the immense stress of having a chronically ill mother addressed. The diagnosis of von Wille-brand disease added another layer of fear, particularly as a family member who had the same disorder experienced life-threatening hemorrhaging during all five of her births. This fear of bleeding out lingered in my mind, shaping my perception of what birth would be like for me.

These early experiences laid the groundwork for the trauma I would face during the birth of my first daughter. However, before I delve into that, I must talk about my sister, who had her own transformative journey with birth. She had four children, but her birth stories were not what one would expect from a mother of four. With her first child, she went past her due date and was induced. This, as is often the case, led to an emergency C-section.

3

For her second child, she was told that a repeat C-section was necessary, so she planned for it, unaware of other options.

Something shifted in her when she became pregnant with her third child. She began researching home birth after cesarean (HBA2C) and decided to pursue a home birth. My initial reaction was one of support but also concern—wasn't this dangerous? Still, I trusted her instincts. She successfully birthed her third child at home and described it as one of the most powerful experiences of her life. Watching her confidence grow and witnessing the profound transformation in her was awe-inspiring.

Her journey sparked my interest in birth work. I was amazed by her strength and intrigued by the idea of helping women have natural births. Her story planted the seeds of what would later become my mission.

When I met my husband at 30, I had long carried the belief that marriage and motherhood weren't for me. This mindset was likely a defense mechanism born from years of being told that my body was broken. I feared the possibility of infertility and the risk of hemorrhaging during childbirth. I convinced myself that not wanting children or marriage would protect me from future disappointment or trauma.

Yet my fascination with the human body persisted. At 19, I became a licensed massage therapist, studying anatomy and physiology with the intent of helping others heal. Although I didn't realize it then, these early steps were guiding me toward the path I'm on today.

When I became pregnant with my first daughter at 37, I immediately dove into research, wanting to understand everything about birth. I enrolled in a doula certification program and became a certified birth doula, postpartum doula, childbirth educator, and lactation counselor. My training was thorough, but in retrospect, much of it was rooted in the medicalized framework that shapes mainstream childbirth education. I was learning about "evidence-based" practices, but this often translated to teaching women how to conform to a system rather than encouraging them to trust their body. Birth, according to this model, was broken down into stages and phases, with an emphasis on external measurements—like contraction timing and cervical checks—rather than internal intuition.

I prepared for my first birth with what I thought was ample knowledge. I had read all of Ina May Gaskin's books, taken a natural childbirth course, and chosen a birth center, which I viewed as a safe middle ground between home and hospital. But as I now know, my first birth was marred by subtle yet significant interventions that ultimately led to a transfer and an emergency cesarean.

My five-day labor, which the system labeled "prodromal" or "false" labor, ended with an epidural due to exhaustion and, finally, a C-section. Reflecting on that birth, I now understand where the process veered off course—where fear, intervention, and lack of trust in my body came into play. Yet, this experience made me the passionate advocate and educator I am today. I share my story openly, not as a cautionary tale, but as an educational tool to show where interference with physiological birth can cause trauma.

In my work as a somatic coach, I help women process their birth trauma by pinpointing exactly where things went awry. Most birth trauma stems from moments where a woman's body was undermined, where interventions disrupted the natural process, or where fear crept in and caused doubt. Understanding the root of that trauma is essential for healing.

Redemptive birth is powerful. After my first birth, I went on to support numerous women in their redemptive births—many of whom had vaginal births after cesarean (VBACs). Witnessing their journeys rekindled my desire for another child and a chance to experience birth as God designed it.

At 40, I became pregnant with my second daughter and knew immediately that I would not set foot in a hospital. I chose midwives whom I trusted and who respected my autonomy. At 41, I had my redemptive home birth—a powerful, unmedicated VBAC. It was the most empowering experience of my life, reinforcing the belief that God designed our bodies perfectly for birth.

The way we talk to ourselves matters. The body believes what we tell it. If we approach birth with fear, uncertainty, or doubt, those feelings can manifest physically. But if we embrace the truth that we are fearfully and wonderfully made, our bodies will respond in kind. Redemption isn't just about having a successful birth after trauma—it's about reclaiming trust in the body's divine design.

So, whether you are a first-time parent, someone who has experienced birth trauma, or someone preparing for a redemptive birth, my hope is that by the end of this book, you will feel empowered, educated, and fully confident in the natural design of your body.

We are all capable of undisturbed physiological birth. Pain tolerance is irrelevant in this context. In fact, the women who often doubt their ability to handle pain without medication are the ones who surrender most beautifully when it comes time to give birth. In the final chapter, I will share a collection of such beautiful birth stories.

CHAPTER TWO

THE PHYSIOLOGY OF BIRTH

*"For you created my inmost being; you knit me together in my
mother's womb. I praise you because I am fearfully and
wonderfully made; your works are wonderful,
I know that full well."*
– Psalm 139:13–14

THE ELEGANCE OF PHYSIOLOGICAL BIRTH

F*ear produces cortisol and tension; cortisol and tension
inhibit oxytocin and create pain. Releasing fear allows
oxytocin to flow; oxytocin promotes relaxation, leading to
a serene, even blissful, birth experience.*

"Healthy mom, healthy baby—that's all that matters." This is
a widely accepted sentiment in our society and is often seen as
the ultimate goal of childbirth. While I certainly agree that the
health of both mother and baby is paramount, it should not be
the only standard to which we aspire. When women choose to
give birth in a hospital, this goal becomes the baseline.

However, the physical well-being of mother and baby post-birth often fails to reflect the emotional and somatic undercurrents that may be present beneath the surface. We witness high rates of postpartum depression, postpartum anxiety, maternal struggles, and even divorce following the birth of children. These phenomena arise partly because we are not adequately educated on undisturbed physiological birth and its profound benefits for mother and baby.

Women, when birthing, are often categorized as "low-risk." Childbirth is as natural a bodily function as urination, sneezing, coughing, or sleeping. We simply birth a baby; it is not a medical procedure that requires excessive management, oversight, or control.

In fact, all mammals experience a natural hormonal rhythm during labor. If you observe animals in the wild—be it a deer, cow, goat, cat, or dog—the first thing they do when entering labor is find a secure, quiet space. This allows them to relax their nervous systems, ensuring a safe birth, free from the threat of predators. This instinctual process is a reflection of the design God has for all mammals, including humans. To feel safe and supported during birth, women must trust the process, and trust begins with knowledge. Understanding the physiological variations of birth outside the constraints of the medicalized framework imposed on women is essential for surrendering to birth.

Much of the trauma experienced during birth does not stem from physical complications but from the loss of a woman's autonomy. Her choices, desires, and birth preferences are often overridden. You might wonder how autonomy can be stripped so easily. Let me explain: when a woman does not know what is normal in pregnancy, childbirth, or even breastfeeding, she becomes vulnerable to external influence. In birth, when we constantly seek validation from others—asking if everything is okay, perfect, or normal—we cease to listen to our bodies. We lose trust in our instincts and disrupt the natural process of birthing, designed to unfold in full faith and surrender.

For example, when an animal begins spontaneous (not induced) labor in the wild, it seeks a quiet, secure space. It does not doubt its ability to give birth. If a predator disrupts the process, the animal's labor hormones shut down, halting the birth so it can move to safety. Once it's secure, labor resumes. This same principle applies to humans. When we enter an environment where we do not feel safe, supported, and unobserved, labor can stall. This is one of the many reasons why home birth is highly recommended.

Mainstream childbirth education is rooted in evidence-based practices often informed by studies conducted in highly medicalized environments, predominantly hospitals funded by pharmaceutical companies. Instead of empowering women to trust their bodies and embrace the undisturbed process of physiological birth, this model teaches women to conform to a system that pathologizes birth. The inherent unpredictability and personal nature of birth cannot be confined to rigid phases or timelines. Rather than focusing on early, active, and transition phases or fixating on dilation, I encourage women to see birth as a series of stages that honor the natural flow of the process.

STAGE 1: LABORING

In undisturbed physiological birth, the baby initiates labor when it is ready. There is no need to nudge the process or attempt natural inductions. Trusting the timing of God and the wisdom of the baby is key. Science supports this process—labor begins at its own pace. Interventions, which will be discussed later in this book, often disrupt this delicate balance and can lead to unnecessary risks and trauma.

I have witnessed women progress from one to ten centimeters

dilated in 45 minutes, or two centimeters to full dilation in just two hours. Labor can start and finish within the span of an hour. This unpredictability is precisely why I do not focus on rigid phases. A woman can be in transition at three centimeters, on the verge of meeting her baby, and experiencing the adrenaline surge that naturally precedes the body's instinct to push. In undisturbed births, the body knows when and how to labor down and begin pushing.

STAGE 2: THE BODY PUSHES

I intentionally use the term "the body pushes" because true physiological birth does not require coached pushing. When undisturbed, women instinctively know when and how to push as their bodies, guided by a natural hormonal cocktail, work in harmony with the baby. In these moments, I have seen women move intuitively, helping their babies navigate through the pelvis in ways that are guided by ancient wisdom.

A very NORMAL thing that happens when a baby is descending into the birth canal is that their heart rate will slow down. This is the "squeeze," and many midwives will just listen to make sure the baby's heart rate returns to baseline between contractions. If you are focused on the sound of a Doppler or monitor, know that this is normal and can scare many women and their partners unnecessarily.

When a baby comes down, they will slowly stretch the cervix. Often, this involves what I call a game of "peek-a-boo." Their head will come down, go back up, come down again, and then go back up. This is designed to slowly stretch you and mold their head so that they can be born. They will do this until, finally, they remain under the pubic bone. From there, they will begin to crown. The head will be born, and often, there may be another rest phase between contractions as the baby makes their rotation for the shoulders to be born.

Being coached to push when a baby hasn't signaled they are ready can lead to the "stuck" that many people speak about. You must listen to your body and allow the breaks. Movement doesn't just stop with labor; you also must move your body if you feel the need during pushing to help the baby navigate their way out. This is not an option if you have received an epidural or are told you can only push in the lithotomy position. (Look into why that position began to be advocated by practitioners... it will blow your mind.)

STAGE 3: BIRTHING THE PLACENTA

The third stage of birth—delivering the placenta—is still a part of the birthing process, though it's often overlooked in hospital settings. In undisturbed physiological births, this phase should not be rushed. I have seen placentas birthed hours after the baby without complications. The body's hormonal response must be allowed to complete its cycle. Low lighting, a calm environment, and uninterrupted bonding with the baby facilitate this final stage of birth.

In many traditional birth settings, the third stage—delivering the placenta—is hurried. Often, medical staff interfere unnecessarily, leading to complications that can affect postpartum bonding, contribute to hemorrhage, or disrupt breastfeeding. Your labor is not truly over until the placenta is birthed, and you must remain attuned to your body during this process, just as you were during labor itself. Oxytocin, the hormone of love and bonding, continues to play a critical role here, helping the uterus contract and the placenta to detach naturally.

Hospital environments tend to focus on time frames, often suggesting that the placenta should be delivered within five to 30 minutes. In my experience, placentas can take significantly longer to be birthed without any adverse effects, provided there are no signs of hemorrhaging (which is often caused by induction or interference in the birth process). In these moments, encouraging natural oxytocin release—by breastfeeding, skin-to-skin contact, or simply being present in a calm environment—can help the body complete this process as nature intended.

Following the birth of the placenta, many hospitals perform what is known as a "fundal massage." This is an aggressive technique to ensure that the uterus contracts fully and can be quite uncomfortable. I strongly advocate for mothers to be educated about this practice and, if necessary, ask to perform the massage themselves. This allows the woman to maintain control of her body post-birth, empowering her to participate in her care rather than being subjected to unnecessary or harsh procedures.

When undisturbed physiological birth occurs, the body's natural rhythms and hormonal responses are allowed to complete their work. Oxytocin, which drives contractions, bonding, and even the production of breast milk, is essential. The flood of this hormone, along with natural endorphins (the body's pain-relieving chemicals), creates a deeply profound and often pleasurable experience for both mother and baby. This is the beauty of physiological birth—it allows mother and child to enter the postpartum period in a state of harmony, bathed in the love and connection that oxytocin fosters. We are to be birthed BATHED IN LOVE!

In contrast, interventions—whether in the form of induced labor, pain-relief medication, or cesarean sections—disrupt this delicate balance, often leading to a cascade of interventions that can result in trauma for both mother and baby. The process becomes mechanical, distanced from the sacred dance that birth was designed to be. I've witnessed firsthand how the introduction of medical interventions disrupts the hormonal flow of labor, which leads to longer recovery times, difficulty in bonding, breastfeeding complications, and often emotional trauma.

Physiological birth is a process that operates best when left undisturbed. The baby, too, plays a vital role. The infant's signals to the mother's body, through the release of prostaglandins, initiate the softening of the cervix. This communication between mother and baby is nothing short of divine design. The baby's descent through the birth canal is orchestrated by a series of innate movements known as the cardinal movements. These movements are the baby's way of navigating the mother's pelvis, whether the baby is head-down, breech, or positioned posteriorly (often called "sunny side up"). The wisdom of the baby, in concert with the mother's body, is awe-inspiring.

As the baby begins to push through the birth canal, the mother will experience a sensation that is often compared to the urge to vomit—but downward. This reflex, known as the fetal ejection reflex, is the body's natural way of expelling the baby without the need for external coaching. Telling a woman to "stop pushing" in these moments is one of the most disruptive things that can be done. The body knows when and how to birth the baby.

Once the baby is born, the umbilical cord, still attached to the placenta, continues to pulse, delivering vital blood and oxygen to the newborn. One-third of the baby's blood is still within the placenta at birth, and the rush of blood into the baby's system is crucial for their immediate health and vitality. This is why delayed cord clamping is essential. Cutting the cord too soon, as is often done in hospital settings, can deprive the baby of this essential blood supply, leading to unnecessary stress or complications. I vividly recall the birth of my second child, whose umbilical cord pulsed for 22 minutes, providing her with oxygen and blood as she transitioned into the world. She didn't take her first breath for over 90 seconds, but because of the support and understanding of the midwives, there was no panic. She was calm, and her pulse was steady as she gently adjusted to life outside the womb.

Rushing this process—cutting the cord prematurely or intervening too soon—can rob both mother and baby of a peaceful transition. Babies sometimes need time to adjust. I've seen instances where babies take several minutes to breathe on their own yet remain perfectly healthy as long as their cord is still providing oxygen. This is why an understanding of physiological birth is so vital for parents and practitioners. The natural process should be trusted, honored, and allowed to unfold without unnecessary interruptions.

Once the umbilical cord ceases to pulse, the placenta will naturally detach from the uterine wall and be birthed. Again, this is not a process to be rushed. The mother's body, still awash with oxytocin, knows precisely how to complete this final stage. In the hospital setting, practitioners often encourage rapid detachment and delivery of the placenta, sometimes resorting to manual removal or unnecessary medications. However, in undisturbed births, the mother's body, given time and space, will expel the placenta without complication.

EMPOWERMENT THROUGH PHYSIOLOGICAL BIRTH

When I educate women about undisturbed physiological birth, I emphasize the wide range of normal variations I've witnessed as a doula. Birth is not something to control; it is a process to surrender to. When women learn to trust their bodies and the process, labor progresses more smoothly and with fewer complications. I also share stories of births that did not follow textbook patterns yet resulted in healthy, positive outcomes.

For instance, I've seen women labor for days with contractions spaced five minutes apart and others who delivered their babies with contractions eight to 15 minutes apart. Hospitals tend to follow a rigid pattern, expecting contractions to be two to three minutes apart before a woman is considered to be in active labor. However, this doesn't account for the variations in how women labor naturally. For some, contractions spaced further apart are perfectly normal. Forcing labor to fit a specific timeline, especially with medications, can create stress and lead to unnecessary interventions. This is where traumatic birth experiences often begin.

Understanding these variations helps women let go of expectations and fears. Trusting in the natural ebb and flow of labor is essential. One of the most important tools during labor is rest. Exhaustion is one of the main reasons women transfer from home or birth centers to hospitals. Early labor is not the time for intense physical activity like curb walking or bouncing on birthing balls. It is a time for rest, to conserve energy for the work ahead. I've helped women take 20-minute naps during the transition phase—right before they push their babies out. Yes, you can nap during labor—if you let go of fear and trust the timing of your body.

A "rest phase" also occurs when the body and baby have reached full dilation but need a moment of calm before pushing. I have seen women completely relax, even fall asleep, during this phase. When they wake, the fetal ejection reflex kicks in, and their body naturally pushes the baby out without any conscious effort on their part. This is the wisdom of physiological birth in action.

INTERVENTIONS AND THE RISKS THEY POSE

The initiation of labor is meant to be spontaneous. Even "natural inductions," such as acupuncture, tinctures, primrose oil, or castor oil, can disrupt the body's hormonal balance. Labor begins when the baby sends signals, releasing prostaglandins to soften the cervix and prepare the mother's body for birth. This process is delicate, and any interference can have consequences. Trusting that the baby and body know when labor should begin is key to allowing the birth to unfold naturally.

After the baby signals readiness by releasing prostaglandins, the brain begins to produce oxytocin. This powerful hormone drives contractions, bonding, and, later, breastfeeding. It is crucial to allow the body to generate and maintain this oxytocin flow. Interfering with the natural process, whether through medications or unnecessary monitoring, can hinder the production of oxytocin, making labor more painful, disrupting the bonding process, and complicating breastfeeding.

The body also releases endorphins—natural pain relievers—which, when combined with oxytocin, can make natural birth an empowering, even joyful experience. The baby and the mother are both flooded with these powerful hormones. Interventions like pain relievers for moms in labor can cut the flow of these hormones to the baby. This leaves the baby to navigate birth while disconnected from mom and can lead to stress. Enjoying the natural, undisturbed process of physiological birth is important. To do this, you must enter into birth empowered and understand your fears so you can face them head on.

CHAPTER THREE

HEALTH AND WELLNESS IN PREGNANCY

"Do you not know that your bodies are temples of the Holy Spirit,
who is in you, whom you have received from God?
You are not your own; you were bought at a price.
Therefore honor God with your bodies."
— 1 Corinthians 6:19-20

When planning for a physiological birth, maintaining a healthy mental and physical state is crucial. I believe there are **five pillars** to focus on during pregnancy: **hydration, nutrition, movement, mindfulness, and meditation/prayer.** Let's explore each one in detail, beginning with hydration, a topic often overlooked in prenatal care. Many women don't understand the "why" behind proper hydration, which makes it easier to neglect. However, once you understand its significance, drinking 90–120 oz. of water daily becomes a purposeful and essential task rather than a burden.

HYDRATION

Hydration plays a vital role in pregnancy. When you are pregnant, your body produces 50% more blood, which requires proper hydration to transport essential nutrients to your baby. Hydration also helps manage issues like constipation by aiding in bowel movements and detoxing the system. Moreover, frequent urination can help prevent urinary tract infections, which are more common during pregnancy.

Another important reason to stay hydrated is to maintain amniotic fluid levels. In late pregnancy, fluid levels are often used as a measure of fetal health, and low levels can be a cause for concern, sometimes leading to unnecessary inductions. Staying hydrated can ensure healthy fluid levels, preventing potential complications. In hospitals, IV fluids are often administered to women who haven't been hydrating enough, but you can take control by drinking water throughout the day. I've seen many women avoid complications, like preeclampsia, by simply staying hydrated.

A common mistake I've noticed is women stopping hydration during the night due to the inconvenience of frequent urination. However, continuing to drink water at night is essential, as your baby still needs hydration, and dehydration can lead to issues like high blood pressure, swelling, and even preeclampsia symptoms.

It's also important to supplement hydration with electrolytes. Adding a pinch of Celtic sea salt and lemon to your water or drinking coconut water can help balance electrolytes and ensure you're retaining essential nutrients. Electrolytes prevent the salts your body needs from being flushed out and support your body's increased demands during pregnancy.

NUTRITION

Just as important as hydration is proper nutrition. Gestational diabetes (GD), a condition where the body struggles to manage insulin levels during pregnancy, is common. Even women who are otherwise healthy can develop GD. Diet plays a critical role in managing blood sugar levels whether you have GD or not.

Unfortunately, many people associate pregnancy with cravings for unhealthy foods like pizza, ice cream, or chips. While occasional indulgences are fine, maintaining a balanced diet is key to both your and your baby's health. Managing GD with a balanced diet, rather than relying on glucose tests alone, is more sustainable. Monitoring how different foods affect your blood sugar through real-time testing can help you make better choices.

For example, seemingly healthy foods like bananas or oatmeal can spike your blood sugar if consumed in excess. Monitoring your body's response to specific foods will help you tailor your diet to avoid unnecessary sugar spikes, which can contribute to preeclampsia or other health issues.

A healthy diet during pregnancy should focus on whole foods, adequate protein intake (at least 60–80 grams per day), and essential nutrients. Magnesium is a particularly important mineral for maintaining blood pressure, improving sleep, and reducing stress during pregnancy. Additionally, prenatal vitamins can help fill nutritional gaps in your diet, ensuring that you and your baby are getting the necessary nutrients.

MOVEMENT

Movement is crucial for maintaining a healthy pregnancy and preparing for the physical demands of childbirth. Pregnancy can be compared to a marathon, so, just like you would for a marathon, you need to train for it. Regular exercise improves circulation, supports healthy blood pressure, and keeps you strong and flexible. Something as simple as walking for 45 minutes a day can make a big difference in how your body feels and functions.

Along with movement, it's important to balance strength with flexibility, especially in your pelvic floor. Strengthening your pelvic floor is important, but so is learning how to release tension and stretch those muscles to avoid tightness during birth. Practices like stretching, chiropractic adjustments, Pilates, and spinning babies exercises can help maintain balance in your body and ensure optimal positioning for your baby.

MINDFULNESS

Mindfulness is the practice of staying connected with your body and being aware of its signals. Pregnancy provides an opportunity to deepen that connection. From the early stages of conception to birth, your body communicates with you, and learning to listen is vital.

Many women tend to ignore bodily signals, such as the need to urinate or feelings of discomfort, often because we've been conditioned to tune out these cues. However, pregnancy offers a chance to reclaim that awareness. By listening to your body during pregnancy, you can become more attuned to what it needs when something feels off so you can better prepare for labor. When it comes time for labor, you'll be more in sync with your body and able to trust its cues without needing constant external validation.

MEDITATION AND PRAYER

Daily meditation and prayer allow you to connect with yourself and God, fostering peace and trust in your body. Taking just five minutes each morning to center yourself and quiet your mind can set the tone for your day. This was something I prioritized during my second pregnancy—taking time to pray for the birth I desired, focusing on my breath, and calming my nervous system.

In our fast-paced, modern society, we often operate in a constant state of stress (sympathetic nervous system), juggling responsibilities, work, childcare, and more. This can take a toll on both you and your baby. By carving out moments of stillness, you can shift your body into a parasympathetic (rest-and-digest) state, which is crucial for your physical and mental well-being.

Taking time to reset and connect to God fosters a sense of peace and trust in your ability to give birth. Setting daily intentions, visualizing a healthy and empowered birth, and having faith in the process will help you cultivate the mental strength to navigate any challenges that arise. It's also important to build an unshakable belief in your body's capabilities, protecting you from any negative influences that might disrupt your trust in the process.

PUTTING THE FIVE PILLARS TOGETHER

By following these practices—hydration, nutrition, movement, mindfulness, and meditation—you can create a balanced, healthy pregnancy and prepare yourself for a beautiful, empowered birth. These elements work together to ensure that you are physically strong, mentally centered, and fully in tune with your body as you journey through pregnancy, birth, and beyond.

CHAPTER FOUR

INTERVENTION AND DISRUPTING NATURE'S DESIGN

"There is a time for everything, and a season
for every activity under the heavens."
– Ecclesiastes 3:1

I frequently discuss on my podcast how choosing a hospital birth, while not inherently dangerous, significantly disrupts the natural processes of labor and birth. Even before you step into a labor and delivery room, multiple interventions—sometimes as many as ten—can alter the physiological birth process.

Let's break them down:

1. **Timing Contractions at Home**. Hospitals and birth centers often instruct you to time your contractions so you know when to leave. The common guideline is five-one-one: contractions five

minutes apart, lasting for one minute, for the duration of one hour. However, this practice takes you out of your body and into your head. I've seen women birth their babies with contractions spaced ten to 15 minutes apart, never reaching the two-to-three-minutes-apart pattern hospitals often expect. By focusing on timing, you move away from being present with your body and, instead, focus on an external metric.

2. **Arranging for Care for Pets or Siblings**. If you have pets or older children, you'll need to arrange for someone to care for them while you're at the hospital. This logistics-driven task pulls you further out of the birth process, shifting your attention to external factors rather than allowing you to remain fully immersed in the progression of your labor.

3. **Physically Leaving Home**. The simple act of leaving your home—your safe, familiar environment—can significantly disrupt your labor. Getting into a car, possibly experiencing contractions while seated uncomfortably, and traveling to a hospital or birth center shifts your focus and can slow the natural labor process.

4. **Checking in at the Hospital**. Upon arrival, the check-in process itself can be unsettling. Bright lights, unfamiliar sounds, and antiseptic smells suddenly surround you. The sterile, impersonal environment of the hospital is a far cry from the peaceful, intimate space you've cultivated at home. This stark change can hinder the flow of labor hormones, such as oxytocin, which are critical for progressing labor naturally.

5. **Meeting Strangers**. When checking in, you're likely to interact with people you've never met before —staff members who don't know you or your birth preferences. Meeting strangers during such a vulnerable and intimate time can cause discomfort, making it harder to remain relaxed and in tune with your body's natural rhythms.

6. **Being Sent to Triage**. Before entering a labor and delivery room, you may be sent to triage. Here, you might be surrounded by other laboring women and asked to fill out forms and answer numerous questions between contractions. This impersonal and clinical atmosphere can further disrupt your labor by pulling you out of the internal, focused state needed to allow the birth process to unfold naturally.

7. **Monitors and Cervical Checks**. To confirm you're in labor, hospitals often rely on external validation, such as continuous fetal monitoring and cervical checks. These interventions tether you to machines, restrict your movement, and reinforce the idea that you need external approval to confirm what your body already knows: that you are in labor.

8. **Meeting Your Obstetrician**. Even if you've built a relationship with your obstetrician during prenatal care, there's no guarantee they will be the one attending your birth. Often, the doctor on call is someone you've never met, introducing yet another unfamiliar face into an already disruptive environment.

9. **Insertion of an IV Port**. Many hospitals routinely insert an IV port upon admission, just in case they need to administer fluids or medication. While you can decline this, receiving an IV during labor can be

uncomfortable and further medicalizes what should be a natural process.

10. **Settling Into Your Labor Room**. Finally, after all the steps above, you enter your labor and delivery room, where new monitors are attached, and you attempt to make yourself comfortable. However, by this point, much of the natural labor process may have already been disrupted, leading to a need for further management and intervention.

These ten steps illustrate how simply choosing a hospital birth —before any medical intervention even occurs—can disrupt the undisturbed physiological birth process. By the time you've arrived, checked in, and settled into the labor room, your body's natural hormone flow, particularly oxytocin, may have been interrupted. As cortisol levels rise due to the stress of the environment, labor often slows, and medical staff may feel the need to intervene to speed things up, initiating what's known as the cascade of interventions.

THE CASCADE OF INTERVENTIONS

A birth plan that includes "no interventions" in a hospital is often unrealistic. It's like expecting a five-star, healthy meal at a fast-food restaurant—it simply doesn't align with the environment. Hospitals are designed to manage birth, and once you choose that setting, interventions are likely. Even with the best intentions, practitioners may push for interventions like Pitocin, cervical checks, and fetal monitoring because they are focused on managing the labor rather than trusting the body's natural process.

One of the earliest interventions, one that sets the stage for many more, is the **due date**. The concept of a rigid 40-week window for birth is arbitrary and can create unnecessary pressure. In reality, the birth window is anywhere from 37 to 42 weeks, and healthy pregnancies can go beyond that range without issue. However, as soon as you pass your due date, many practitioners start discussing induction, which often leads to a cascade of further interventions.

When we try to control the timing of birth—whether through due dates or induction—we interfere with the baby's natural readiness to be born. This can disrupt bonding, breastfeeding, and postpartum recovery, as the natural hormonal process has been altered.

THE ROLE OF SCANS AND TESTS

Interventions don't just occur in labor; they begin during pregnancy with routine tests and scans. For example, the **gestational diabetes test** can often produce false positives, especially when relying on the glucola drink. Instead, I recommend pricking your finger after meals to monitor your blood sugar levels in real-time. This approach is far more informative and provides a better understanding of your body's unique responses.

Similarly, **ultrasounds** are often overused. While they can be helpful, particularly for identifying issues like placenta previa, too many scans introduce unnecessary anxiety. Misjudging a baby's size, for instance, can lead to unnecessary discussions of C-sections or other interventions. This is also true for concerns about the baby's position. Rather than attempting to manually turn a breech baby through invasive procedures, we should recognize that breech is a natural variation of birth and can be safely managed if practitioners are trained in these techniques.

THE HARM OF CERVICAL CHECKS

Cervical checks, particularly those performed before labor has even started, are a common but often unnecessary intervention. Such checks cannot predict when labor will begin, yet many women are led to believe that they provide important information. For example, you could be dilated to four centimeters at 34 weeks and still not go into labor until 41 weeks, or you could be completely closed and go into labor the next day.

Cervical checks during labor are equally problematic. They interrupt the natural hormone flow, and the results can often disappoint or discourage laboring women. Being told you are only three centimeters dilated when you feel like you're deep into labor can cause doubt, which, in turn, can stall labor. I've seen women progress from one to ten centimeters in under an hour, defying the expectations set by cervical checks. When women aren't subjected to these checks, they remain more connected to their bodies and can surrender to the process without external validation.

PITOCIN AND EPIDURALS: THE UNSEEN IMPACT

One of the most common interventions in hospitals is **Pitocin**, a synthetic form of oxytocin. Unlike natural oxytocin, which works in a feedback loop with the brain and body, Pitocin bypasses this system, leading to harder, more painful contractions without the accompanying emotional benefits of natural oxytocin. It increases the likelihood of requesting an epidural, which further disrupts the body's natural processes.

Pitocin and epidurals are often used together, creating a cycle of intervention that leads to more risk and less control. Pitocin speeds up labor, but because it creates more intense contractions, women often need an epidural to cope with the pain. However, the epidural can slow labor, leading to the need for even more Pitocin to stimulate contractions. This cycle can result in complications like fetal distress, the need for assisted delivery with instruments, or even a cesarean.

ARTIFICIAL RUPTURE OF MEMBRANES

Another seemingly small intervention with big consequences is the **artificial rupture of membranes** (breaking the water). The amniotic sac plays a crucial role in helping the baby position itself during labor. When the water is broken artificially, the baby may shift into an undesirable position, making it more difficult for it to navigate the birth canal. This often leads to further interventions, like forceps or vacuum-assisted deliveries, which could have been avoided if the water was allowed to break naturally.

When your water breaks, the MOST IMPORTANT thing is not inserting things into your vagina so you don't increase your risk of infection. However, if a woman's water breaks naturally, most practitioners want to perform cervical checks multiple times, adding risk where there was none. I have seen women go 72 hours after their water has ruptured before going into labor. They were hydrating, resting, getting checks on the baby, and trusting their body would start when it was time. The clock of 18–24 hours is not a box you should put yourself into if you are not getting cervical checks.

TRUSTING THE PROCESS

Interventions aren't inherently wrong, but they should be used judiciously. Each adds a layer of risk and can disrupt the delicate balance of hormones that drive labor. When an intervention is suggested, it's important to ask questions (B.R.A.I.N.):

- What are the **benefits** of this intervention?
- What are the **risks**?
- What are the **alternatives**?
- What does your **intuition** tell you?
- What happens if you do **nothing**?

In many cases, doing nothing—allowing labor to unfold naturally—is the best course of action.

CHAPTER FIVE

CHOOSING YOUR BIRTH TEAM

"Walk with the wise and become wise,
for a companion of fools suffers harm."
– Proverbs 13:20

Whether you envision birthing with just your partner or plan to have a midwife for a home birth, possibly along with a doula, friends, or family, one of the most crucial decisions you will make is choosing who to include in your birth space. These people can profoundly influence the outcome of your birth, and while familiarity is comforting, what matters most is their knowledge and understanding of undisturbed physiological birth. Anyone present who harbors fear or doubt about the birth process can unintentionally project that energy onto you, which could disrupt the natural flow of labor.

For example, if you wish to have your mother or sister in the room, consider their personal experiences and beliefs about birth. Have they given birth themselves, and if so, how do they view it? A single, misguided comment at a critical moment can cause you to doubt yourself, especially during a time when you are most vulnerable due to the heightened hormonal activity in your body. Surround yourself with people who trust in your ability to birth and who support your desire for a natural, undisturbed experience. Your birth team should reinforce your confidence, not undermine it.

It's important to remember that while your birth team will support you, they are not the ones giving birth—you are. However, their influence can either uplift and empower you or instill doubt. This is why it's crucial to choose people who align with your vision and understand that intervention is not always necessary.

On my podcast, I often talk about the concept of the "bait and switch." This can happen with any practitioner, from obstetricians to midwives. The bait and switch occurs when a practitioner initially seems fully supportive of your birth plan, but as the pregnancy progresses, they introduce fear-based care or drop hints that suggest they may not be as supportive as you thought. Spotting this shift early on is key because you don't want to find yourself scrambling for a new practitioner late in your pregnancy.

I don't believe practitioners do this out of ill intent. The reality is that our medical culture is steeped in fear when it comes to childbirth, particularly in the United States. Many doctors and midwives have been conditioned to believe that birth requires management and intervention. They are accustomed to working with women who may not be fully educated about undisturbed physiological birth or may not be maintaining the healthiest pregnancy. This instills doubt in their minds about every woman's ability to birth naturally. For this reason, they often approach birth with skepticism, which can manifest as a lack of trust in the natural process.

It's also important to note that the health of the mother

largely dictates the outcome of the pregnancy and the birth. This is why I stress the importance of proper nutrition, hydration, movement, and supplementation throughout pregnancy. When you take care of your body, you are laying the foundation for a healthy, intervention-free birth. A practitioner who sees that you are doing everything to maintain your health may have more confidence in your ability to birth naturally.

Although midwives are generally more supportive of natural birth than obstetricians, they, too, can have fears associated with the process. However, their fears often stem from concerns about whether a mother is doing everything she can to maintain a healthy pregnancy—whether she is staying hydrated, nourishing herself properly, and so on. Their fear is less about the birth itself and more about the mother's ability to sustain a healthy pregnancy, which ultimately reflects in the birth.

So, how do you choose the right practitioner, midwife, doula, or anyone else you want present at your birth? I've created a list of key questions to ask when interviewing potential members of your birth team:

1. **How do you feel about me going into spontaneous labor, even if this happens after 42 weeks?** The response to this question will be very telling. As I've mentioned, the concept of a rigid due date is arbitrary, and many women can go past 42 weeks and still have a perfectly healthy birth. If your provider's response is anything less than full support of your body's natural timing—as long as both you and the baby remain healthy—then they likely do not fully support undisturbed birth and may push for induction as you approach or pass 42 weeks.

2. **How do you feel about vaginal breech birth?** Breech birth, while less common, is still a natural

variation of normal. However, many practitioners are not trained in how to assist with vaginal breech deliveries, often opting for cesareans instead. If your provider has not taken the time to learn about breech birth or is uncomfortable with it, this indicates that they may not fully respect the nature of undisturbed physiological birth.

3. **How do you feel about having minimal to no ultrasounds?** Ultrasounds, like any other medical intervention, come with both risks and benefits. While they can be useful in certain cases, such as identifying placenta previa, they are often overused. Many obstetricians will perform between five to ten scans throughout a pregnancy, which is unnecessary and can lead to anxiety rather than reassurance. If you prefer fewer ultrasounds, make sure your provider respects this and understands your desire to rely more on your body's intuition.

4. **How do you feel about a VBAC (vaginal birth after cesarean)?** VBACs are often portrayed as risky, but in reality, they carry no greater risk than a vaginal birth for a first-time mother. The language around VBACs is often manipulative, with terms like "trial of labor after cesarean" (TOLAC) being used to undermine a woman's confidence. If your provider does not fully support VBACs or if they suggest it is a "trial," this could indicate that they are not the right fit for you.

5. **How do you feel about delaying cord clamping and immediate skin-to-skin contact?** Delayed cord clamping allows the baby to receive the full benefit of the blood from the placenta, while immediate skin-to-skin contact promotes

bonding and helps regulate the baby's temperature and breathing. A provider who understands the importance of these practices will support you in delaying interventions such as weighing and measuring the baby until after this critical bonding period.

6. **What is your protocol for delivering the placenta?** The third stage of labor—delivering the placenta—is still an integral part of the birth process. Many providers will want to speed up this stage, often using Pitocin to hasten the delivery of the placenta. However, the placenta can take time to naturally detach, and forcing the process can disrupt the body's natural hormonal flow. A provider who respects the natural timeline of birth will not rush this stage and will allow you to deliver the placenta in your own time.

It's essential to ask these questions and observe how your provider responds, both in words and body language. Their answers will give you insight into whether they truly support undisturbed birth or if they are likely to push for intervention when the time comes.

Now, let's shift the focus to doulas. A good doula is not only an emotional and physical support person during labor but also a source of knowledge and empowerment throughout your pregnancy. Doulas help calm fears, educate you on the birth process, and provide practical support during labor, such as reminding you to hydrate, helping you relax, and encouraging you to trust your body. They play a critical role in helping you avoid exhaustion, which is one of the most common reasons for hospital transfers during home births.

Doulas also serve as advocates for you, ensuring that your

birth plan is respected, particularly during the vulnerable moments after birth when you may not be able to advocate for yourself. For example, you may ask your doula to protect the third stage of labor, making sure no one pulls on the cord or rushes the delivery of the placenta without your consent.

In some cases, women may choose to have what is known as a "free birth," birthing without the presence of any medical professionals and relying solely on their own intuition and support from their partner. While free birth is not for everyone, if you feel empowered and confident in your ability to birth without intervention, it is a valid and beautiful choice. No one should shame you for choosing this path, as it is your birth, your baby, and your decision.

Birth is a sacred rite of passage. It deserves the same level of attention, care, and respect that we often give to other major life events, such as weddings. Too often, we follow the birthing paths of those around us without truly understanding or preparing for the experience. By taking the time to educate yourself and carefully select your birth team, you can create a birth that is not only safe but also empowering, honoring the natural design of birth as God intended.

When you surround yourself with people who trust the process, honor your autonomy, and support your birth plan without judgment or fear, you set the stage for a truly beautiful, undisturbed, physiological birth.

CHAPTER SIX

THE WAYS LABOR BEGINS

*"As you do not know the path of the wind, or how the body
is formed in a mother's womb, so you cannot understand
the work of God, the Maker of all things."*
– Ecclesiastes 11:5

As women approach their due date, I start receiving many texts: *How will I know when labor begins? Is this my mucus plug? Is this normal?* They often send pictures or describe sensations, seeking outside validation. As their doula, I reassure them that what they're experiencing is typically normal, but I also remind them that the most important thing they can do is ignore early signs of labor and get some rest. When labor *does* kick into gear, they will need that energy.

A common question I hear is, *How will I know if it's real labor?* The way Hollywood portrays labor has misled many—water breaking suddenly, a rush to the hospital, and then screaming in the delivery room. In reality, that's not how labor usually unfolds. If your labor starts with your water breaking, known as **PROM** (premature rupture of membranes), which happens in about 10–13% of births, there's no need to panic. You can still rest, hydrate, and treat it as though labor hasn't fully begun. You'll want to make sure the fluid is clear and without a foul smell or an unusual color. If everything checks out, your next step is to go back to bed. Hydration is crucial if your water breaks since the body replenishes amniotic fluid.

I've seen too many women hastily induced for "low fluid" when, often, simply drinking water with electrolytes would solve the problem. So, if your water breaks, keep hydrating and rest—two of the most vital tools in your arsenal.

If your labor begins with your water breaking, sensations typically start within 12–24 hours. This is your chance to rest, sleep, or keep yourself distracted with light household tasks. Studies suggest women with lower vitamin C levels are more likely to experience **PROM**, though I can't confirm this as a doula. However, I've noticed that women who follow vegan, vegetarian, or pescatarian diets tend to have labor start with their water breaking, which may relate to lower protein intake or lack of collagen, commonly found in animal products. That's just my observation.

One crucial tip: after your water breaks, don't put anything into your vagina. Doing so increases the risk of infection, especially if you get cervical checks, which many hospitals push for. Avoiding them will nearly eliminate your risk of infection.

TYPICAL LABOR ONSET

Most often, labor begins quietly, often in the middle of the night when your body's labor hormones peak. While labor can start at any time of day, I usually get calls from 11 p.m. to 4 a.m. This is when the body and mind are most relaxed, allowing labor to initiate. There's something powerful about how labor begins when we're at rest—our bodies know when we're ready, and that readiness often coincides with our sleep.

When this happens, the best thing to do is try to get more rest. Keep a heating pad nearby for comfort, sip water, and focus on your breath. It's common for fear to creep in, which is natural. Having a supportive partner or doula at this point can help calm your nerves. Try to go back to sleep—labor tends to take its time, so there's no need to rush to "do" something like bouncing on a birth ball or taking a curb walk. Instead, focus on relaxing your muscles, unclenching your jaw, lowering your shoulders, and easing tension in your face. This simple mindfulness can help your body progress through labor naturally.

One great tool for early labor is what I call the "dilation station": the toilet. Sitting on the toilet relaxes the pelvic floor, and it's a place where we're naturally accustomed to releasing tension. Imagine labor as similar to having diarrhea. If you were experiencing that sensation, you wouldn't be panicking about timing your bowel movements or asking if something was wrong. You would ride the sensation, knowing your body is working as it should. Labor is no different—it's about surrendering to what your body already knows how to do.

PRODROMAL LABOR

Labor might also begin, especially for first-time moms, as prodromal labor—often mistakenly referred to as "false labor." While frustrating, prodromal labor is not useless; it's your baby trying to get into a better position for birth. It might cause contractions that feel very real and intense, softening the cervix but not necessarily progressing into active labor right away. When prodromal labor occurs, things like chiropractic adjustments or spinning babies exercises can help get the baby into a more favorable position.

Often, prodromal labor is a sign of emotional or mental tension—unreleased fear can block labor from progressing. I've seen this firsthand. When a mother releases that fear, sometimes with a good cry, labor can shift into full gear. Emotional release is just as vital as physical adjustments in preparing for labor to progress naturally.

RELAX AND TRUST THE PROCESS

When labor starts, it can be tempting to time contractions and seek validation that "this is it." However, doing so pulls you out of your body and into your head. Trust that your body knows what to do. If you experience contractions ten minutes apart, and then labor seems to stop for two hours—take a nap. Your baby might be resting, and you should follow suit. When labor picks back up, you'll be more prepared for the intensity of the next wave.

The key is to rest, stay hydrated, and not worry too much about timing. Everyone's labor is unique. Some women lose their mucus plug weeks before labor begins; others might experience a "bloody show" closer to the start of labor. Whether your water breaks early or you're experiencing intense sensations, trust that your body and baby are working together in perfect harmony.

Labor begins differently for every mother and baby. You may lose your mucus plug early, you may see blood, or your water may break. These are all variations of normal. The most important thing is to trust your instincts, relax, and surrender to the process. Whether your labor lasts for days or happens in just a few hours, it's all part of your unique journey. The key to labor is surrender—rest, hydrate, nourish your body, and trust that everything is unfolding as it should. You can do this.

CHAPTER SEVEN

BREAKING DOWN THE FEARS

"For the Spirit God gave us does not make us timid,
but gives uspower, love, and self-discipline."
— 2 Timothy 1:7

F ear often finds its way into the birth journey long before labor begins. It can stem from personal experiences, societal narratives, or generational trauma. Recently, at a mother's blessing ceremony for one of my doula clients, we engaged in an exercise where the expectant mother was encouraged to voice her fears aloud so we could symbolically burn them away. She expressed a profound realization: to fully embrace the birth portal, she also needed to acknowledge the death portal. Birth and death are intimately linked, she said, and to surrender completely and step into that void—to retrieve her baby with full faith—she needed to trust entirely in God.

This powerful acknowledgment highlights a significant divergence between medical establishments and spiritual trust. The medical system often instills a reliance on technology and inter-vention, whereas embracing faith means trusting in the natural design of our bodies and the divine process of birth.

THE FEAR OF TEARING

One of the most common fears surrounding childbirth is the fear of perineal tearing. At the mother's blessing, a woman asked if the expectant mother's husband had begun perineal massages to prevent tearing. I immediately interjected, assuring her that such measures were unnecessary. Tearing can occur during birth, and that's okay; our bodies are designed to heal. In undisturbed physi-ological births, significant tearing is rare. Most women experience minimal tearing because they are attuned to their bodies, empowered, and have no fear-induced tension in the pelvic floor.

Tension and fear can contribute to tearing. When a woman is fearful of pushing her baby out, she may unconsciously tighten her pelvic muscles, increasing the likelihood of tearing. Often, traumatic tearing stories come from births that involved interven-tions or took place in hospitals. Interventions like epidurals can disconnect women from their bodily sensations, leading them to push against contractions without feeling them fully. Instrumental deliveries using forceps or vacuum extractors can exacerbate the risk of severe tears.

In contrast, home births typically involve minimal tearing. Women are more likely to listen to their bodies, change positions as needed, and push instinctively, reducing the risk of significant perineal trauma. Even if a tear occurs, the body is remarkably resilient and capable of healing.

THE FEAR OF PAIN

Pain is another pervasive fear in childbirth. However, reframing the concept of pain as one of intensity can transform the birth experience. Labor is undeniably intense, but it doesn't have to be painful in the traditional sense. By embracing the sensations and viewing them as powerful waves bringing you closer to meeting your baby, you can reduce fear and tension.

Fear triggers the release of cortisol, a stress hormone that can inhibit the production of oxytocin—the hormone responsible for uterine contractions and the progression of labor. When oxytocin flow is hindered, labor can slow down, leading to interventions that may not have been necessary otherwise.

Educating and empowering yourself before conception or during pregnancy can help you break down these fears. Understanding the physiology of birth and trusting in your body's innate abilities can alleviate anxiety about pain. Embracing the intensity of labor as a natural and purposeful sensation allows you to surrender to the process, facilitating a smoother birth experience.

GENERATIONAL TRAUMA AND SOCIETAL FEAR

Many fears are rooted in generational trauma and societal narratives. Women who grew up hearing traumatic birth stories—from forceps deliveries to episiotomies—may internalize these fears. The medicalization of birth in past decades has removed agency from women, leading to an increase in experiences that are more traumatic than transformative.

Birth is meant to be a rite of passage—a sacred ceremony where both a child and a mother are born. When fear dominates this experience, it can overshadow the profound beauty and empowerment that birth offers. Trusting in the divine design and embracing faith can help counteract the fear instilled by medicalized narratives.

THE FEAR OF LOSING THE BABY

The fear of losing the baby is profound and deeply personal. Miscarriages and stillbirths, while relatively rare, are part of some women's stories and can cast a long shadow of fear over subsequent pregnancies. Medical professionals may inadvertently exacerbate this fear by emphasizing worst-case scenarios or using fear-based language.

For instance, in hospital settings, I've witnessed practitioners use phrases like "dead baby" to pressure women into interventions. This manipulation exploits a mother's deepest fears, pushing her to make decisions that may not align with her desires or best interests.

It's crucial to acknowledge these fears but also to trust in your body and the natural process of birth. Maintaining open communication with supportive practitioners who respect your autonomy can help alleviate unnecessary anxiety.

THE FEAR OF UTERINE RUPTURE IN VBACS

For women considering a vaginal birth after cesarean (VBAC), the fear of uterine rupture is often amplified by medical professionals. While uterine rupture is a serious concern, it occurs in less than 1% of VBAC attempts. Despite this low risk, the fear is used to justify continuous monitoring and interventions that can, paradoxically, increase stress and hinder labor progression.

Medications used to induce or augment labor, such as Pitocin, can increase the risk of uterine rupture. Ironically, the interventions intended to prevent complications can sometimes contribute to them. Choosing a supportive environment—often outside of the hospital setting—where you can labor undisturbed may reduce these risks.

THE FEAR OF HEMORRHAGING

Postpartum hemorrhage is another significant fear. While hemorrhaging can be life-threatening, understanding its causes and taking preventative measures can mitigate anxiety. Many hemorrhages result from interventions that disrupt the natural third stage of labor—the delivery of the placenta.

In undisturbed births, the placenta typically detaches and is expelled naturally, aided by the continued flow of oxytocin, especially when the baby is placed skin to skin and begins breastfeeding. Immediate cord clamping, aggressive uterine massage, or pulling on the umbilical cord can interfere with this process, increasing the risk of hemorrhage.

Maintaining a calm environment, allowing the mother and baby uninterrupted bonding time, and trusting in the body's ability to complete the birth process can help prevent complications.

THE FEAR OF PASSING THE DUE DATE

Fixating on due dates can create unnecessary stress. A due date is an estimate, not an expiration. Only about 5% of babies are born on their estimated due date. It's normal for labor to begin anywhere from 37 to 42 weeks of gestation. Going past 40 weeks does not inherently indicate a problem.

External pressures—from practitioners eager to schedule inductions to well-meaning friends and family checking in—can heighten anxiety. Trusting in your body's timing and maintaining open communication with your care provider about your preferences can alleviate this fear.

THE FEAR OF A LARGE BABY

Concerns about birthing a large baby often lead to discussions of induction or cesarean delivery. However, estimations of fetal size via ultrasound can be off by up to two pounds. Fear of shoulder dystocia (where the baby's shoulder becomes lodged behind the mother's pelvic bone) is commonly cited, yet this complication is relatively rare and can often be managed with positional changes during birth.

Our bodies are designed to birth the babies we grow. The size of the baby is usually proportional to the mother's pelvis and ability to birth naturally. Trusting in this design and having a care provider who supports this trust is crucial.

THE FEAR OF ADVANCED MATERNAL AGE

Women over the age of 35 are often labeled as "geriatric" pregnancies, a term that can instill fear. While certain risks do increase slightly with age, overall health is a more significant determinant of pregnancy and birth outcomes than age alone. A healthy, active woman in her 40s can have a perfectly normal pregnancy and birth.

Rejecting labels that don't serve you and focusing on your well-being can empower you to approach birth with confidence rather than fear.

EMBRACING FAITH AND TRUST

Breaking down fears requires a combination of education, self-reflection, and trust—in your body, your baby, and the birth process. Surrounding yourself with supportive individuals who reinforce this trust can make a significant difference.

Remember that fear and faith cannot coexist. By choosing to

focus on faith—whether spiritual, faith in your body's capabilities, or both—you create a mental and emotional environment conducive to a positive birth experience.

Embrace the intensity of labor as a powerful force bringing your baby into the world. Release tension and surrender to the process. Your first act of motherhood is to trust in the natural design, allowing you and your baby to experience birth as it was intended—bathed in love, empowerment, and joy.

CHAPTER EIGHT

EMBRACING NATURE AND SURRENDER

"Be still, and know that I am God."
– Psalm 46:10

Having explored the essence of undisturbed physiological birth, the importance of choosing a supportive birth team, and the necessity of breaking down fears, we arrive at the crux of the matter: embracing nature and surrendering to the innate wisdom of our bodies. This chapter delves into why trusting in God, nature, and our intuition is paramount in childbirth and beyond.

TRUSTING IN NATURE AND GOD

As a doula, educator, and lactation counselor, my practice is grounded in the belief that we must trust our bodies and the natural processes designed by God. In a world saturated with information on how to parent—from sleep training methods to feeding schedules—it's easy to become overwhelmed and disconnected from our inner guidance. I encourage mothers to tune into their bodies and instincts. If a particular approach feels right deep within your being, embrace it. This is not about shaming different choices; it's about fostering a harmonious bond between mother and child as nature intended.

If interventions like epidurals or elective inductions at 38 or 39 weeks resonate with you, then this perspective might not align with your journey. This discourse is intended for those who wish to reconnect with the natural design of childbirth and motherhood, recognizing that we are perfectly made to conceive, carry, birth, and nurture our children.

THE EARLY STAGES: CONCEPTION AND PREGNANCY

Trusting nature extends beyond labor and birth; it begins in the conception phase and continues through pregnancy. Many women rely on ovulation strips, apps, or basal body temperature readings to predict conception, often leading to misconceptions about their pregnancy timeline. For instance, with my first daughter, I conceived around day 24 or 25 of my cycle, not on the presumed day 14 indicated by ovulation predictors. Consequently, dating ultrasounds showed a two-week discrepancy.

Imagine if I had sought an ultrasound at what I thought was the eighth week of pregnancy, only to find no detectable heartbeat or visible embryo due to the miscalculated timing. Sadly, many women face this scenario and are prematurely advised to terminate what could be a perfectly healthy pregnancy. I've witnessed women who believed they were eight or nine weeks along, only to discover later that they simply had smaller yet healthy babies at full term.

This highlights the importance of patience and trust. Instead of rushing to medical interventions or relying solely on technology, consider waiting a few more weeks or forgoing unnecessary ultrasounds altogether. Listen to your body; it knows when it is pregnant. If there are genuine concerns, your body will signal when medical attention is needed.

CHOOSING THE RIGHT SUPPORT

Embracing nature doesn't mean rejecting all medical assistance or forgoing professional support. Opting for a home birth with a qualified midwife provides the best of both worlds. Midwives can monitor your baby's health, perform necessary checks like Doppler heart rate monitoring, and order blood work to ensure your well-being. They respect the natural process while being prepared to assist if complications arise.

It's essential to understand that choosing a natural, undisturbed birth doesn't equate to recklessness or neglect. It's about recognizing that you are the primary agent in your birthing experience. No one can birth your baby for you. You must do the work of labor, but having a supportive, knowledgeable practitioner by your side can provide reassurance and assistance when necessary.

THE IMPORTANCE OF DELAYED CORD CLAMPING AND IMMEDIATE BONDING

When a baby is born, the transition from the womb to the outside world is profound. In some births, babies may not breathe immediately upon emergence—a normal variation in the spectrum of birth experiences. The umbilical cord, still pulsating with life, continues to deliver oxygen-rich blood, stem cells, and vital nutrients essential for the baby's initial moments.

In hospital settings, the standard practice often involves cutting the cord quickly and whisking the baby away for assessments, which can interrupt this critical physiological process. By delaying cord clamping and allowing the baby to remain on the mother's chest, we honor the natural design. Skin-to-skin contact regulates the baby's temperature, heart rate, and breathing, facilitated by the mother's body—a phenomenon no external warmer can replicate accurately.

THE IMPACT OF ENVIRONMENT AND SUPPORT ON BIRTH

The environment in which you give birth significantly affects the hormonal interplay essential for labor and postpartum recovery. Oxytocin, the "love hormone," thrives in settings where the mother feels safe, unobserved, and supported by familiar faces. This hormone not only drives labor contractions but also fosters bonding and reduces the risk of postpartum hemorrhage.

Surrounding yourself with people who trust in your ability to birth naturally amplifies this hormonal harmony. Fear and stress can disrupt oxytocin production, leading to complications that might necessitate interventions. By creating a peaceful, supportive environment, you align with the body's natural processes.

THE JOURNEY OF SURRENDER

Pregnancy and childbirth are profound exercises in surrender. From conception, where we cannot see the intricate developments within our wombs, to labor, where we must release control and let our bodies lead, we are called to trust deeply. This surrender extends into motherhood, where we learn to attune ourselves to our babies' needs without constantly seeking external validation.

Surrendering requires faith—in God, nature, and ourselves. It's about recognizing that while we cannot control every aspect of this journey, we can choose how we respond. By embracing gratitude, prayer, and meditation, we strengthen our ability to let go of fears and anxieties, opening ourselves to the transformative power of birth.

BREASTFEEDING: CONTINUING THE PATH OF TRUST

Breastfeeding is another area where surrender and trust are essential. Often, women find it to be more challenging than birth because it involves two people learning a new skill together. Society inundates us with messages that can undermine our confidence: doubts about milk supply, pressures to supplement with formula, and unrealistic expectations about infant behavior.

In these moments, returning to the question, "What would I do if I were in nature?" can be grounding. In a natural setting, a mother would nurse her baby whenever the child showed signs of hunger or distress, without questioning her body's ability to provide. Trusting that your body can nourish your baby is vital. Recognizing that fussiness or frequent feeding can be normal aspects of growth spurts or developmental leaps helps alleviate unnecessary worry.

THE RIPPLE EFFECT OF TRUST

By mastering the art of surrender and trust during pregnancy and birth, you set the foundation for a more intuitive approach to parenting. This trust allows you to respond to your child's needs with confidence and calmness, fostering secure attachment and emotional regulation.

Imagine a generation raised by parents who are deeply attuned to their children's needs, who trust their instincts over societal pressures, and who prioritize connection over convenience. The impact on societal well-being would be profound.

OVERCOMING SOCIETAL CONDITIONING

Breaking free from societal conditioning requires conscious effort. We are often told to seek external validation for every aspect of our health and parenting, leading to a disconnection from our intuition. Medical check-ups, while valuable, should not replace our innate ability to sense when something is amiss.

It's important to discern when interventions are truly necessary and when they stem from a culture of fear and mistrust. By educating ourselves, seeking supportive communities, and reaffirming our faith in the natural design, we reclaim our autonomy and empower ourselves as mothers.

RECLAIMING OUR DIVINE DESIGN

Embracing nature and surrendering to the process of childbirth is a radical act of trust in a world that often promotes control and intervention. By aligning with the way God and nature have designed us, we honor not only our bodies but also the sacred journey of bringing new life into the world.

This path is not about rejecting medical care outright but making informed choices that resonate with our deepest instincts and values. It's about recognizing that we are fearfully and wonderfully made, equipped with everything we need to birth and nurture our children.

As you continue on this journey, remember that you are not alone. Countless women have walked this path before you, tapping into the profound strength and wisdom that comes from trusting in the natural design. Embrace this wisdom, surrender to the process, and witness the transformative power it brings to your life and the lives of your children.

CHAPTER NINE
VBAC IS LOW RISK

"I can do all things through Christ who strengthens me."
– Philippians 4:13

I know far too many women who have had unnecessary C-sections, and they often question whether they can have a vaginal birth after a cesarean (VBAC). The answer is absolutely yes, you can. A vaginal birth is generally much safer than a C-section, and the recovery process is significantly less taxing. Much of the trauma and unnecessary complications that arise from C-sections could be avoided if more women were offered the opportunity for a vaginal birth. That's why it's essential to break down the fear surrounding VBAC and learn to trust your body's natural ability to birth the baby you are growing.

Too often, emergency C-sections are performed for reasons like "the baby got stuck" or "the baby was too big." However, these reasons are frequently inaccurate. Understanding what truly happened during your first birth is key to moving forward with confidence. You need to fully process your first birth experi-ence—only then can you trust your body and your baby as you prepare for a VBAC. This is crucial because, if you continue to doubt your body or question whether you truly needed a C-section the first time, those fears will take over during your next labor.

I love working with women to heal their birth trauma. It's a beautiful transformation to witness when they start to believe in the possibility of giving birth as nature intended. My goal isn't to give false hope but to restore their autonomy, to offer them the choice that should have always been theirs: the option for a vaginal birth after a C-section.

Unfortunately, some places categorize VBAC as "high risk," but it should never be considered that way. I've already discussed the minimal risk of uterine rupture, which is less than 1% (0.5%, to be exact). You are just as safe, if not safer, having a VBAC at home. Even if your first birth ended in trauma—whether through a C-section, obstetric violence, or a rapid, overwhelming delivery—educating and empowering yourself can change every-thing for your next birth. When a woman is truly empowered, she can fully embrace the powerful hormonal process of birth, bathed in oxytocin, that undisturbed physiological birth creates.

However, many VBAC stories I read still carry remnants of trauma because the birth took place in a hospital environment. These stories usually start with something like, "My OB broke my water to speed things up, so I wouldn't get too tired. I'm so grateful." However, when you introduce interventions like breaking the water or inducing labor, you add unnecessary risks and begin the cascade of interventions that often lead back to the same complications women want to avoid.

Inductions during a VBAC are particularly problematic because they force the body to do something it may not be ready for. This can lead to stronger, more frequent contractions that require additional interventions, such as Pitocin. For women who have had uterine surgery, like a C-section, Pitocin is contraindicated. Administering Pitocin increases the risk of uterine rupture, the very complication that medical professionals claim to fear most during a VBAC.

Some women have experienced rare complications like placental abruption or placenta previa, and while these can be legitimate reasons for a C-section, it's important to remember that just because something happened once, it does not mean it will happen again. You have to release the fear that history will repeat itself and trust in your body's ability to birth normally.

Breech presentation is another factor that leads women to have unnecessary C-sections. Breech birth is a variation of normal, not an automatic emergency. However, in many states, it's illegal for midwives to deliver breech babies at home, even if they are trained to do so. This is why the work of professionals like Dr. Stuart Fischbein, who teaches practitioners how to safely deliver breech babies, is so vital. Women should not be forced into surgery simply because a provider is uncomfortable with a breech delivery.

Fear plays a massive role in unnecessary interventions. If we focus on fear, we manifest the very things we are afraid of. Instead, we must pray, visualize, and focus on the positive. You can have a beautiful VBAC, but it requires letting go of fear and trusting your body, your baby, and God. This is where true redemption lies. I have been privileged to witness many women achieve this redemption through their HBACs (home birth after cesarean), and it is one of the most powerful experiences.

It's important to understand that VBAC is not a "trial of labor," as many hospitals call it. You are laboring—you are birthing, and you are doing it. You will have your redemption. The opportunity for a VBAC should always be offered to women, and if the medical system doesn't support it, there are other paths like free birth or finding a midwife who truly believes in your body's ability to birth naturally.

Every woman deserves to experience the power of a physiological birth, free from unnecessary interventions. We should teach girls from a young age about their bodies, their menstrual cycles, and how birth works. This knowledge will help them trust their bodies when the time comes instead of relying on a medical system that profits from the idea that women's bodies are broken.

If you have had a C-section, it's normal to question your body and lose some trust in its ability to birth, but you can regain that trust. God gave you the wisdom to know your body. The fear that keeps women from embracing their VBAC options is part of a system that profits from keeping them in the dark. However, once you are empowered with knowledge and trust in your body, your fear diminishes, and you can reclaim your power.

Obstetricians don't often witness undisturbed physiological births. They see the transfers and the emergencies, so, of course, they think home birth is dangerous. But imagine if more obstetricians could witness the beauty and power of a hands-off, natural birth. It would challenge their fears and perhaps open their minds to the true design of birth.

C-sections are necessary about 4% of the time, not the 30–40% we see today. Too many women are being told that they "need" a C-section when, in reality, they could safely have a vaginal birth. You owe it to yourself and your future baby to explore the possibility of a VBAC. Find a supportive practitioner, labor at home for as long as possible, and advocate for yourself in the hospital if that's where you feel safest. You can have the birth you desire.

Remember, redemption doesn't stop at birth. A successful VBAC often leads to a smoother breastfeeding journey, as your body and baby are in harmony. The flood of oxytocin and other hormones after an undisturbed birth helps establish breastfeeding, bonding, and physical recovery in a way that C-sections often disrupt.

I've witnessed women have three C-sections and then go on to have a beautiful VBAC at home. You are not broken. You were made perfectly, and your body is capable of birth. Whether this is your first baby or your fifth, you deserve to experience birth as it was designed—undisturbed, empowered, and in line with the divine wisdom of your body. Embrace your redemption. Trust in your body, trust in your baby, and trust in the process God created.

CHAPTER TEN

FAITH OVER FEAR

"Now faith is confidence in what we hope for and assurance
about what we do not see."
− Hebrews 11:1

This verse from Hebrews speaks directly to the heart of pregnancy, birth, and motherhood. In the beginning, we cannot see the moment of conception. We might guess that a sperm cell met an egg on a certain day, but we don't truly know the precise second that new life was created within us. From the very start, we seek outside validation, starting with the date of our last period, often leading to what's known as a "dating ultrasound." This is supposed to confirm the gestational age of the baby and predict the due date. However, even this is only an estimate and cannot pinpoint the exact moment or day our baby will arrive.

In fact, only 4% of babies are born on their predicted due date. That means 96% of the time, the baby arrives earlier or later, outside of this so-called "normal" range that the medical system relies on. Despite this, there's often pressure to keep you as close to that arbitrary due date as possible.

I remember vividly when I went for my dating ultrasound. I thought I was nine weeks pregnant, but the ultrasound technician measured my baby and said, "According to this, you're seven weeks and two days." I felt disappointed. I thought I was further along, closer to the so-called "safe zone" of pregnancy. That moment marked the beginning of me doubting my body's intuition. I believed I knew when I had conceived, but the machine told me otherwise. This external validation, this measurement, suddenly carried more weight than my inner knowing.

I shared this story with my midwife, and she assured me that dating ultrasounds are highly accurate. I felt a tug in my spirit—a knowing deep within me—that this wasn't true, yet I let that external validation overshadow my faith in my own body.

This happens often. A woman might believe she's eight or nine weeks pregnant when she goes for an ultrasound, but they can't find a heartbeat, or the baby is measured as being much smaller than expected. Sometimes, the heartbeat simply isn't detectable with the available technology, especially if the baby is smaller or if you are earlier along than you thought. Fear creeps in. We're told that the baby might not be viable, and some women are offered medications to "help" expel the baby from their womb.

In these moments, I tell women, "Wait four more weeks. If it turns out that it is a true miscarriage, I will come and hold that space with you. We will honor your baby's life in a sacred way. I or your partner will be there to support you." Often, if we trust our bodies and have patience, we see that all is well. Fear drives so much of this process, especially the fear of not knowing.

From the very beginning—right when we pee on that stick or miss our period—we seek validation that the baby inside us is healthy, that it's growing and thriving. However, this external validation doesn't truly ease the fear. The only thing that does is faith: faith in your body, faith in God, and faith in the process.

Birth and death are closely connected. You have to accept both if you are to truly surrender to the birth process. I'm not suggesting everyone should have a completely unmonitored pregnancy, but I do believe that ultrasounds in the first trimester are often unnecessary. If you need validation, have your HCG or progesterone levels checked instead. There are natural ways to support these levels, especially if you have thyroid or other health concerns.

If you do choose to have an ultrasound, do it with joy and curiosity, not fear. However, make sure you are fully informed about the potential effects of ultrasound on your body and your baby. Do your own research and empower yourself to make the decision, not because someone else told you to but because you are making an autonomous, educated choice. The foundation of this process is faith over fear.

The practice of faith begins even before conception. Trusting your body and believing that God will bring a baby to your womb allows you to calm and regulate your nervous system. Get your levels tested if that helps. Adjust your diet and care for your body—but always remember that faith is what will carry you through the uncertainties of pregnancy, birth, and motherhood.

Fear is pervasive in our culture, especially when it comes to birth: fear of miscarriage, fear of complications, fear of what happened to someone else. However, living in a state of fear robs you of the peace and joy that pregnancy can bring. Fear raises cortisol levels, which negatively affects your body, your baby, your hormones, and, ultimately, your birth experience. Replace that fear with affirmations, declarations of faith in your body's abilities.

Here are some affirmations you can hold on to:

- My body and my baby are working together.
- I am strong and capable of giving birth.
- My body knows exactly what to do, and I trust it.
- I surrender to the sensations of birth, knowing they bring me closer to meeting my baby.
- Each contraction is powerful, just like me.
- I breathe, I relax, I trust.
- I was made for this.

Writing these affirmations and surrounding yourself with them throughout your pregnancy is like creating a prayer or a vision board. The more you internalize these beliefs, the more your body and mind will align with them. They will become second nature. Faith will take root, and fear will no longer have a place in your heart.

Having faith over fear isn't just a mantra for pregnancy and birth—it's essential for your journey as a parent. There will be countless moments of uncertainty, but faith in your body, your baby, and God will carry you through. Birth is a natural, physiological process designed to work perfectly when we trust it and don't allow fear to interfere.

Ninety-nine point nine percent of the time, birth goes right when left undisturbed. The key is keeping your mind and spirit focused on trust, calm, and faith. Through education, empowerment, and connecting with God, you can overcome the fear that might try to take hold.

Affirmations, deep breathing, prayer, and connection to your body's innate wisdom will carry you through labor. Keep reminding yourself:

- My body has everything it needs to birth my baby.
- I am confident in my ability to give birth with joy and love.
- I trust the process.
- I trust my body and my baby.

These are not just words—they are truths that, when spoken into existence, have the power to transform your experience. Having faith over fear means surrendering to the process, knowing that no matter what happens, you are capable, strong, and divinely supported.

Faith will always be stronger than fear, and when you fully embrace faith, you will find a peace that surpasses understanding.

CHAPTER ELEVEN
BREASTFEEDING AND LEAPS

*"For you will nurse and be satisfied at her comforting
breasts; you will drink deeply and delight
in her overflowing abundance."*
– Isaiah 66:11

I've often wondered whether I should record podcast episodes about breastfeeding. Every woman's breastfeeding journey is so different, and there are countless tools, pieces of advice, and varying opinions that can easily derail what could otherwise be a beautiful and positive experience. As someone who has helped many women, I know that, just like birth, breastfeeding can offer women a path to redemption—a chance to have the experience they truly desire. Too often, I hear stories of women who "just couldn't produce enough," whose supply "dried up," or whose babies "weaned early." While these things happen, they are not inevitable. Many of these experiences can be linked to how women approach their breastfeeding journey from the start.

In our modern world, we tend to deviate from nature's design in many aspects of motherhood, including breastfeeding. For instance, we place an enormous focus on creating nurseries—separate rooms for the baby to sleep in—before the baby is even born. However, this separation disrupts the natural process of bonding and breastfeeding. When the baby is placed in another room, we miss their cues. Breastfeeding is about connection, tuning in to your baby's needs, and helping them develop a strong latch and the strength to breastfeed effectively. It's a learning process for both the mother and baby.

Breastfeeding is often challenging and frustrating in the early stages. However, I tell my clients that by six weeks postpartum, they'll likely feel confident, empowered, and grateful that they persevered through those initial struggles. The key is having a strong support system. You need someone who believes in you and your ability to breastfeed—someone who won't quickly suggest formula or encourage longer sleep at the expense of feeding. While it's true that babies need rest, understanding the fundamental principle of breastfeeding—supply and demand—is critical. Breastfeeding works on a simple concept: the more your baby feeds, the more milk you produce.

In the early days of breastfeeding, the baby consumes colostrum, not milk. Colostrum is a thick, nutrient-rich substance packed with antibodies, and babies only need a small amount to fill their tiny tummies. Many mothers panic when they don't see milk right away, especially if the baby seems fussy or refuses to latch for long. This leads to doubt about supply, but it's important to remember that colostrum is all the baby needs in those first few days.

When I work with mothers seeking a "breastfeeding redemption," I start by asking about their birth experience. Birth and breastfeeding are deeply interconnected. A mother's ability to produce milk and establish a good breastfeeding routine is often affected by how the birth unfolded. Did she have trauma? Was there a C-section? Was Pitocin used after birth? These factors can all play a role in milk production and breastfeeding success.

Many women struggle with supply issues because they aren't feeding their babies frequently enough in those early days. The recommendation is to feed every two to three hours—not to impose a strict schedule but to help regulate the baby's blood sugar and ensure they are getting enough nourishment. Sleepy babies, especially those born after long labors or with interventions, may need to be woken up to feed. Allowing a baby to sleep for extended periods, especially in the first few weeks, can signal your body to produce less milk.

The first few weeks are critical for establishing your supply. Ideally, you should aim for eight to ten feedings per day or more if your baby is cluster feeding during growth spurts. The breast operates like a faucet—constantly filling up between feedings. If you don't drain it regularly, your body absorbs the milk, potentially leading to clogged ducts or even mastitis. Keeping the breasts emptied every two to three hours signals your body to continue producing the milk your baby needs.

In my work as a lactation counselor, I focus on helping women set up their milk supply. If the supply is there, other challenges—like problems latching or discomfort—can often be worked through. A healthy supply is the foundation for a successful breastfeeding journey. If you wait too long between feedings, especially at night, your supply may diminish, which is when supplementation might become necessary.

Nighttime feedings are crucial. While it's tempting to let your baby sleep longer at night, it's during these times that they're often the most fussy or going through growth spurts. At night, babies are also more likely to cluster feed, which is essential for boosting your supply. This is why the idea of separate nurseries, while popular, can be counterproductive. Your baby needs to be near you at night, whether in a bedside bassinet or safely co-sleeping, so you can respond to their cues.

Breastfeeding is not just about nourishing your baby—it's also about regulating their body temperature, heart rate, and even blood pressure. Skin-to-skin contact is crucial, especially in the first few days. The baby's tiny stomach can hold only small amounts of colostrum, and frequent latching ensures they get what they need. If there is any disruption to this process—whether through separation at birth or other complications—it's important to pump or hand express to stimulate milk production.

As I often tell mothers, the first few days are challenging. Babies cry and fuss, cluster feed, and sometimes seem insatiable. This is all part of the process. Their fussiness doesn't mean you aren't producing enough milk. It's natural for them to lose some weight in the first week, but by the second, they should be back to their birth weight. Trust the process, trust your body, and trust your baby. Breastfeeding is not meant to be easy, but it is meant to work.

Cracked nipples, engorgement, and discomfort are common, but they don't necessarily mean something is wrong. If breast-feeding is excruciatingly painful, seek help from a lactation consultant to ensure the latch is correct. Some women have sensitive skin, and some experience issues like vasospasm, which can cause pain, but these challenges can often be resolved with the right support.

Just like birth, breastfeeding is a process of surrender. You're learning a new skill alongside your baby, and there will be moments of frustration. Your baby might be fussy, seem gassy, or cry inconsolably, but this doesn't mean you aren't producing enough or that something is wrong with your milk. Colic is often misunderstood and, in many cases, can be relieved with chiropractic care or craniosacral therapy.

Remember, breastfeeding is a dynamic process, and your baby will experience growth spurts and developmental leaps that affect their feeding patterns. These leaps happen every couple of weeks in the newborn phase—at two weeks, four weeks, six weeks, and so on. During these times, your baby might cluster feed more, fuss, or seem unsettled. This is normal, and they are simply using the breast for comfort as well as nutrition.

At four months, there is often what is called the "four-month regression," but it's actually a progression in your baby's development. Their brains are growing rapidly, and they're beginning to see the world more clearly. Their sleep patterns may change, and they may become more fussy or restless at night. This doesn't mean something is wrong—it's a natural part of their growth. Trust the process.

Breastfeeding is not just about feeding your baby. It's about bonding, comforting, and regulating your baby's nervous system. It's a divine design, and every challenge you face in those early weeks is temporary. If you need help, reach out to someone who supports your breastfeeding journey—whether it's a lactation consultant, a friend, or even me. You are capable, and your body is perfectly designed to nourish your baby.

CHAPTER TWELVE

POSTPARTUM REST AND RECOVERY

"Come to me, all you who are weary and burdened,
and I will give you rest."
– Matthew 11:28

In Korean culture, it's believed that how a woman is cared for in the first 40 days postpartum will affect her health for the rest of her life. This wisdom holds significant importance because so many women, especially mothers, walk through life dysregulated, fatigued, and disconnected. Much of this can be traced back to how they were supported—or not supported—after giving birth.

The question often arises: do you need a lot of money for a good postpartum recovery? The answer is no, but in countries like the United States, where postpartum recovery is often rushed due to the pressures of returning to work, the time needed for true healing is rarely given enough value. This oversight leads to increased rates of postpartum anxiety, depression, and breast-feeding struggles, all of which can impact mother and baby long term.

THE IMPORTANCE OF MATERNAL HEALTH

"Healthy mom, healthy baby" doesn't end when the baby is born. The health of a mother deeply influences how well she can care for her baby. It's vital to recognize that the postpartum period is a crucial part of a woman's overall well-being.

After preparing for pregnancy, birth, and breastfeeding, many mothers find themselves forgotten in the postpartum phase. This period, often referred to as the "fourth trimester," is one of the most challenging phases in a woman's life. She is healing from childbirth—whether from a vaginal birth or a C-section—while also learning to care for a new life. Unless she has a constant support system, postpartum recovery can feel isolating and over-whelming.

PRIORITIZING POSTPARTUM CARE

When setting up a baby registry, instead of focusing on unnecessary items, consider prioritizing resources for postpartum care. Set up a postpartum fund to hire help, such as a doula or postpartum specialist, who can assist with tasks like cooking, cleaning, laundry, and even holding the baby so you can shower or rest. These practical forms of support are often far more valuable than expensive baby gear, especially in the first six months of a baby's life.

Think of it like planning for a wedding—where thousands of dollars are spent for one day. Birth is a much more significant event in a woman's life, yet the expenses for postpartum care are rarely prioritized. A natural birth with a midwife might cost between $5,000 to $7,000, while a doula or postpartum doula might charge between $800 to $2,000. Investing in proper care during the postpartum period is just as crucial as any other major life event.

If you want to go all out with postpartum care, find someone who offers "first 40 days" services. This often includes providing warm soups, herbal teas, massages, and other healing remedies that help the mother recover fully. During this time, it's essential to rest. Ideally, the only times you should be getting up are to shower or use the restroom. Your pelvic floor and body are still recovering, and rest is vital to proper healing.

WEEK-BY-WEEK RECOVERY: REST AND NOURISHMENT

After an undisturbed natural birth, many women feel an adrenaline rush and a sense of invigoration, which can lead them to overexert themselves too soon. This is why there's a saying: **week one in the bed, week two around the bed.** In the first week, mothers should rest as much as possible. By the second week, you can move around more but still avoid strenuous activities like going up and down stairs, cooking, or doing household chores. If someone can bring you meals or help with day-to-day tasks, let them. The more you slow down and prioritize nourishment and rest, the faster and more complete your recovery will be.

THE VALUE OF SLOWING DOWN

In today's world, it's hard to slow down. However, this period of forced stillness is where deep intuition, bonding, and self-awareness are born. During the postpartum phase, it's crucial to let go of unnecessary distractions. Emails can wait. Social media posts can wait. What matters most is being present with yourself and your baby.

When visiting a new mother, remember: **don't take the baby from the mother.** The mother and baby need to remain together as much as possible, skin to skin. If you're a mother and worried about someone holding your baby when you're not comfortable, stay in your PJs or keep the baby skin-to-skin. This makes others less likely to grab the baby and keeps the mother-baby bond intact.

Set clear boundaries before the baby arrives. Let people know that no one should kiss the baby. Newborns are especially vulnerable to infections, including cold sores that may not be visible on an adult but could be deadly for a newborn. Protect your baby by keeping them close, following nature's design.

SUPPORT FOR THE MOTHER

After the birth, it's the partner's role to nourish and support the mother. The calmer and more loved a mother feels, the better she will be able to care for her baby. Encourage friends and family to set up meal trains or offer to help with household chores instead of just visiting the baby. If you have trouble asking for help, now is the time to overcome that. Asking for support, setting boundaries, and focusing on rest will ultimately benefit you and your baby.

MANAGING VISITORS

Limit visitors in the first two weeks. Postpartum anxiety often stems from mothers doing too much too soon, and hosting visitors is a major contributor, as it can disrupt rest, delay breastfeeding cues, and cause a mother to overexert herself. If someone insists on visiting, don't hesitate to give them a task like doing the dishes or folding laundry. You are not obligated to entertain anyone, and the focus should be on your recovery and bonding with your baby.

PROTECTING YOUR HEALTH

Listen to your body. If your postpartum bleeding increases or you feel faint or dizzy, it's a sign that you're doing too much. Hydration is also essential during this time. Stay nourished with nutrient-rich foods, supplements, and plenty of water to support your recovery and milk supply.

EDUCATION AND EMPOWERMENT ON SENSITIVE DECISIONS

Topics like vaccines and circumcision are personal and require careful, informed decision-making. While I don't give advice on these topics, I encourage every parent to educate themselves thoroughly. Understand the science, do your research, and make decisions from a place of empowerment, not fear.

THE CONNECTION TO RECOVERY

The deeper connection you build with your baby through rest and presence will impact your entire parenthood journey. Many issues, like postpartum depression, anxiety, and bonding difficulties, arise when the postpartum period is rushed or neglected. The importance of nurturing yourself and fully resting in these early days cannot be overstated. Going against the natural design of rest and recovery often leads to long-term disconnection, stress, and health challenges for mother and child.

By respecting the process, embracing rest, and taking care of yourself during this sacred period, you are setting the foundation for a healthier, more peaceful future for you and your baby. **Never underestimate the importance of postpartum recovery.**

CHAPTER THIRTEEN

BIRTH STORIES

*"From birth I have relied on you; you brought me forth
from my mother's womb. I will ever praise you."*
— Psalm 71:6

When I was pregnant with my first child, I read *Ina May Gaskin's Guide to Childbirth*. It's such a wonderful book filled with beautiful, empowering birth stories. Reading and hearing about positive birth experiences can be incredibly uplifting. Such stories remind us that our bodies are designed to give birth, and knowing that other women have had incredible, natural births can inspire hope and confidence.

However, far too many traumatic birth stories are circulating, and it only takes one fearful story to plant unnecessary doubt in a mother's heart. That doubt can stay with her throughout her pregnancy, influencing her mindset during birth. It's important to listen to empowering birth stories, but I also believe there is value in sharing stories that include some trauma, not because we need to dwell on fear but because we need to understand how fear, intervention, and a lack of support can impact the birth process —and, most importantly, how to heal from it.

That's why I've chosen a range of birth stories to share here —some that involve trauma, some that are completely redemptive, and others that are straightforward. Each story has its lessons, and in those with trauma, I'll break it down from my perspective as a doula. Trauma often stems from interfering with the natural, undisturbed physiological birth process. This is how I approach trauma work: breaking down the experience to understand what caused it and how to release it.

This chapter isn't just about sharing stories. It's about offering hope and redemption, especially for mothers who have experienced trauma and are seeking healing through their next birth. You can have a redemptive, powerful birth, but you have to break down the fear, acknowledge the trauma, and move toward full trust and surrender.

MY BIRTH WITH ADELINE

My first birth story is deeply personal. It was with my daughter, Adeline. I was 37 when I got pregnant, and for many years, my husband and I had agreed that we weren't going to have children. We loved the idea of traveling and living a carefree life together, but something inside me shifted, something I didn't fully understand until after her birth.

When I found out I was pregnant, I was excited and ready. I threw myself into learning everything I could about natural childbirth. I watched *The Business of Being Born* and took natural childbirth courses, including hypnotherapy, and I felt prepared. I chose to birth at a birth center, thinking it was a good balance between the hospital and home birth. This is a common choice for women who aren't quite ready to have a home birth. In hindsight, I wasn't entirely prepared for what was to come.

The birth center I chose was 13 minutes away from my house and accepted health insurance, but only my labs and ultrasounds were covered. It should have been a red flag, but I didn't question it at the time. About 50 midwives worked there, and I rotated through as many as I could during prenatal visits to increase the chances of having a familiar face at my birth. At 37, I was treated as high-risk, but they managed it gently enough that it didn't feel overwhelming.

In one of the centering classes, we were taught childbirth education. Now, I don't recommend receiving childbirth education from the same place you'll be birthing. They tend to teach you how to be a good patient rather than how to avoid intervention. I liked all the midwives I met, but looking back, I can see that some of the language they used planted seeds of doubt in my mind.

At one of my appointments, a midwife commented on my weight gain, saying it was too much. I remember feeling judged. I had been eating so clean, so healthy, yet that one comment made me feel like I was doing something wrong. From that point on, instead of focusing on growing a healthy baby, I started watching my diet as if I were trying to lose weight.

There were other red flags, like when I asked if they could use a fetoscope instead of a Doppler at 28 weeks. The midwife seemed hesitant but agreed. They had cautioned against excessive Doppler use in class, but when I asked for a more natural alternative, they weren't very accommodating. This was a small thing, but it added to a growing sense of unease.

Another issue was the glucose test. I had expected the more natural fresh test, but instead, I was handed a bottle of glucola. I resisted, knowing it was full of chemicals, but they insisted that it was "dye-free" and safe. Feeling pressured, I drank it despite my instincts telling me otherwise. I later failed the test and was diagnosed with gestational diabetes. This was the start of a cascade of unnecessary interventions. From that point on, I had to see a maternal-fetal medicine specialist every two weeks.

At 30 weeks, the world was hit by the COVID-19 pandemic, and everything changed. My husband wasn't allowed to attend appointments, and the constant fear of the virus added stress to my pregnancy. I was eating poorly because we were limiting grocery trips, and my once-healthy routine fell apart. Fear took over my entire pregnancy journey.

By the time I reached labor, I had what I call "prodromal labor"—four or five days of exhausting, on-and-off contractions that left me sleep-deprived and anxious. When I finally went to the birth center, I wasn't far enough along, so they sent me home with a shot of Nubain to help me sleep. This cycle repeated itself until, exhausted and discouraged, I was finally admitted, but at that point, I was so worn out that I couldn't progress naturally.

The midwife offered to break my water, and things intensified quickly. I remember thinking, "I'm almost there," but I was only seven centimeters and exhausted. That's when I was told about the "torture position" to speed things along. I gave up and transferred to the hospital. After more interventions, including Pitocin, I ended up with a C-section due to fetal distress caused by infection. I had received about seven cervical checks after my water had broken.

Adeline was born healthy, but I was left traumatized by the experience. It took me 12 weeks to begin questioning what had gone wrong. That's when I dove deep into understanding birth and what had happened to me. I began working with women who had gone through similar experiences and helped them find healing. I became the "VBAC doula" and found immense joy in helping women achieve their vaginal births after cesarean.

But I wanted my own redemption. I wanted to experience birth as it was designed—undisturbed, natural, and powerful. This desire grew as I witnessed more and more women reclaim their births, and I knew that my next birth would be different... and it WAS!

AGAINST ALL ODDS: 43.1/HBAC/BREECH

This next story truly changed my understanding of birth. It showed me why we can't always assume what's going on inside a woman's body or why a baby might be doing something unexpected. This birth was a testament to the unpredictability of birth, the power of trust, and the resilience of the mother. It's a story of redemption—a home birth after a C-section, just like mine, but with even more faith and surrender.

Her first birth journey took her to 42 weeks. She had mentally and physically prepared for a home birth and hired a midwife who was willing to support her at 42 weeks. Once she reached that point, she tried all the natural methods—primrose oil, castor oil, and tinctures—to encourage labor. After three days, there was still no sign of progress, so she transferred to the hospital for an induction. In Texas, licensed midwives are free to go beyond 42 weeks if they feel comfortable, unlike in other states where gestational limits legally bind midwives.

She underwent an induction process, but 36 hours later, her cervix had only dilated to four centimeters, and her baby was floating high. The doctors told her that her baby wasn't engaging, possibly due to a pelvis that was "too small" or a cervix that had "failed to progress." She ended up with a C-section.

When I met her six weeks postpartum, she was struggling with breastfeeding, as many C-section moms do. The lack of proper postpartum support had made the early days hard on her. Her body was recovering from the long induction, but we worked together to help her successfully breastfeed for over 18 months. During that time, I encouraged her to trust her body's ability to birth naturally if she had another child, though I could sense her resistance to the idea. I kept reminding her that she could have a VBAC if she wanted it.

When she got pregnant again, I was thrilled when she called me to be her doula. I could hear the excitement in her voice when she said, "I'm going for a home birth!" I was also pregnant at the time and preparing for my own home VBAC, so we shared the journey. We worked through her fears, especially the fear of going past 42 weeks again.

As her birth approached, around 39 weeks, we met to talk. "Your due date's next week," I said, "but let's not focus on that, right?"

She agreed, laughing as she said, "I've already set my due date to 42 weeks."

I smiled. "Why not 43, for your sanity?" We knew her body's timeline could extend past 42 weeks, so we prepared for that possibility.

When she reached 41 weeks, her midwife sent her for an ultrasound to check on the baby. Everything looked perfect. We kept waiting, and the night before she hit 42 weeks, she texted me that she felt like labor might be starting. There were cramps, and the baby was moving a lot. I was excited—maybe she'd avoid going beyond 42 weeks after all!

The next day, however, when she went for another ultrasound, the baby had flipped into a breech position. Now, here we were: 42 weeks, a home birth after a C-section, and a breech baby. I reassured her that babies can flip anytime they want, even late in pregnancy. There's always room if they choose to flip. I reminded her that we had a midwife who specialized in breech births and fully trusted her ability to birth her baby naturally. Still, I could see how this challenged her faith in her body, especially after the trauma of her previous C-section.

The next couple of days were mentally tough for her. She prayed, surrendered, and listened to her Christian hypnobirthing app to stay calm. At 43 weeks, she texted me again, saying she thought she was in prodromal labor. I went to her house and helped her relax and rest. Her toddler was running around, distracting her, so I suggested that her mother take the toddler to a nearby hotel to give her and her husband the peace they needed.

That night, with her toddler at the hotel, she finally went into labor. The next day, she texted me: "I think this is it!" I rushed over, excited to support her. She labored beautifully and fully surrendered to the process. When the midwife arrived, we all sighed with relief as she confirmed that the baby had flipped back to being head down.

Even though breech is a variation of normal, it was one less thing to work through, and I could see the calm wash over my client. The midwife sat with her, holding space, while my client requested a cervical check. I expected her to be far along—perhaps eight or nine centimeters—but the check showed other-wise. My client could tell from the midwife's expression that she wasn't as far as she hoped. I told her, "It doesn't matter. I think you're going to have this baby in a couple of hours."

The baby was still high, which had been the issue in her first labor, leading to her C-section. This time, however, the situation was different. We weren't going to rush anything. The midwife and I both trusted the process. Sure enough, after a few more hours, her baby engaged and was born beautifully.

This birth reinforced for me that a cervical check does not tell the whole story. A baby will engage and come when the time is right. Despite it being a home birth after a C-section, at 43 weeks and one day, with a baby that had flipped breech at 42 weeks, this mother had still had an incredible birth. Her confidence remained unshaken, and her birth is a story I will share again and again to show how birth can exist outside the "box" that we so often place it in.

FETAL EJECTION

This next mama was a first-time home-birth mom. She and her husband had taken my courses, and we met monthly to break down any fears they had. We went over how birth works, especially how undisturbed physiological birth is meant to unfold. The two of them soaked it all in, and I could tell that this mother truly believed in everything we discussed. She trusted the natural process and her body.

They were also a Christian couple, and their faith was central to their journey. We had to break down her mother's birth trauma. Her mom, like many of our mothers, had one of those dramatic stories—tearing from "one hole to the next," a horrific, painful experience that had left her scarred emotionally and physically. She wouldn't wish it on anyone. I had to break that narrative down and explain why things had happened the way they had. Her mother had experienced obstetric abuse in a hospital, but this mama was birthing at home. She wasn't going to face that kind of abuse. She would be free to listen to her body's cues, breathe her baby down, and allow her body to work as it was designed to.

I told her over and over again, "No one will coach you to push. You won't be told to hold your breath and count to ten. You will simply listen to your body and allow it to labor your baby down and out." These words stuck with her. She embraced them fully.

She was 38 weeks and five days when she had an appointment with her midwife at 10 a.m. After providing a urine sample, her midwife noted that her protein levels and blood pressure were a little high. The midwife called me to let me know that another midwife was on her way to do a blood draw to ensure that it was safe for her to give birth at home.

Immediately, I called the mother to check in. "Did you hydrate?" I asked. She admitted that she hadn't had any water yet that morning despite waking up feeling extremely thirsty. "Your urine was probably pretty concentrated, then," I pointed out. "I need you to drink more water and try to urinate a few times before they come to take your labs. Your high blood pressure could be due to dehydration." I also reminded her about the magnesium the midwives had recommended. She followed the advice, hydrated, and took her magnesium, and I went to be with her, as she was becoming worried about a potential transfer to the hospital.

We sat together, discussing her options if a transfer was recommended, and I reassured her that she always had the choice to say no. A little while later, the blood test results came back perfect. As we talked, she mentioned that she was experiencing sensations that felt like early labor.

When I called the midwife to share the results and discuss what was happening, the midwife dismissed it. "It's not labor, Emmy. It's probably just her uterus being angry because she's dehydrated." This reminded me of the dismissive response I had received from a birth center during my first birth. Since then, I'd learned not to discount a mother's intuition, so I hung up the phone and said to the mother, "You might be in labor. Why not get some rest?"

That night, right before 39 weeks, she called me at 10 p.m. "They're getting really intense and patterned," she said. She believed she was in labor. Who was I to question a first-time mom at 39 weeks saying she's in labor? I grabbed my bag and went to her. When I arrived, she was in full surrender to the sensations, laboring beautifully. She was doing everything she needed to do —breathing, focusing, and letting her body lead.

I suggested we move to the room where she planned to birth. "Why don't we draw a bath and create a peaceful space for you to labor?" I asked.

She looked at me, a little unsure, and said, "Do you think I'm really in labor?"

I smiled. "Yes, you are in labor. No one can tell you if you are or aren't. If you feel you're in labor, then you're in labor."

She went deeper into her labor process. Six hours later, she was in her bathtub, riding each wave with grace and intensity. As we were all quietly waiting for the crowning moment, suddenly, her baby *flew* out of her. I had never seen anything like it. It was a perfect example of fetal ejection. She didn't push her baby out; her body did. Everything we had talked about—the breathing, the surrendering—had stuck with her on a deep, somatic level. She had faith and trusted her body, and the two worked in complete harmony.

She also proved that her body was perfectly fine despite the concerns about preeclampsia and the earlier dismissals of her labor. It wasn't preeclampsia. It wasn't false labor. It was just her body doing what it was designed to do. She had the confidence of a seasoned home-birth mother, and I truly believe that's why her labor was just six hours and that baby came flying into the world.

It was a powerful thing to witness.

BRING ON THE PAIN

I remember when this mom reached out to me. She lived in my neighborhood and had seen that I was known as the VBAC doula of Austin. My name had come up in a couple of different Facebook groups, and when she realized we lived right around the corner from each other, she contacted me. Surprisingly, we had never met before, though our first two children were the same age, and both of our births had ended in C-sections. We could have known each other this whole time.

She and her husband met with me, and we began working together to break down her fears. We also started walking around the neighborhood weekly. She had decided to attempt a VBAC (vaginal birth after cesarean) at a hospital, and while I kept encouraging her to consider a home birth, she wasn't quite there yet. Since I was still working as a doula in hospitals at the time, I decided to empower her to labor at home for as long as possible, minimizing the chances of unnecessary intervention.

One of the first things she told me was, "I'm just so scared of the pain." With her first birth, she had been so afraid of the pain that when the first few mild contractions hit, she and her husband packed their bags and rushed to the hospital. Once there, she immediately asked for an epidural, which set the stage for a cascade of interventions. She was induced, and the process didn't go well. The baby's heart rate dropped, and she ended up with a C-section. Her breastfeeding journey suffered, and she didn't want to repeat that experience.

"I don't ever want to go through what I went through the first time," she told me. "I want to have a VBAC. I've been listening to VBAC podcasts and stories, and I want that." She confessed that she was worried about handling the pain. "I've never even broken a bone. I stub my toe and cry like a baby. How will I handle labor?"

I reassured her, saying, "You will have your VBAC. But we have to keep your mind strong. Your body can handle it."

We spent a lot of time breaking down her fears one by one. I would also prepare her for her doctor appointments. "Okay, this is what they're going to say at week 37," I'd tell her, and when she'd come back from her appointments, we'd walk and talk about what happened.

"You were right," she'd say. "That's exactly what they said."

In week 38, I warned her, "At 39 weeks, they're going to suggest induction. They'll tell you that induction will make your VBAC easier, but it's false."

Sure enough, at her 38-week appointment, the induction conversation came up. She stood her ground, saying, "No, thank you."

When 39 weeks finally arrived, I got the call. "I think it's happening," she said. I was thrilled and rushed to her house—it took me only two minutes to get there. She was laboring beautifully on her birth ball, listening to music while she waited for her parents to pick up her daughter. Her husband, a firefighter, was doing his best to support her, and everything was going well. Her contractions were patterned, about three minutes apart, and growing stronger.

Once her parents picked up her daughter, we decided it was time to go to the hospital. When we arrived, we checked into triage, and by the grace of God, a midwife was there. The midwife requested a cervical check, but my mama was empowered. "No, thank you," she said. "I'm in labor—you can see that."

"Well," the midwife replied, "we can't admit you to labor and delivery without a check." My client stood firm, declining again, so the midwife offered an alternative: "If your water breaks, we can admit you."

I said to my client, "Your water is probably going to break soon, so there's no need to worry." I added, jokingly, "Or you'll just have the baby right here in triage, and that's okay, too!"

Her husband, who could see through the gaslighting that so often happens in hospitals, was growing visibly annoyed with the process. As I applied counterpressure on her back and held a heating pad in place, I heard a splash on the floor. I peeked out from behind the curtain. "I think your water just broke," I said.

"I think I have to go to the bathroom," she replied. "I feel like I need to use the restroom."

I smiled. "Well, sometimes that's just the baby's head."

She insisted, however, and sure enough, her bowels were emptying. This is a common occurrence right before a baby is born. The intensity of her contractions increased significantly once her water had broken.

Finally, we were admitted to a labor and delivery room. As the mother entered transition, I could see how deeply she was immersed in the experience. She was fully present, working through each contraction with strength. The OB came in several times to offer her an epidural, but each time, she refused. "Just remember," the OB said, "there's no reward for doing this unmedicated."

That comment irked me, but my mama stayed strong and true to her goal. When it came time to push, she delivered her baby in just five or six pushes.

Her breastfeeding journey began beautifully, and about a year later, on her son's birthday, she said something that stuck with me: "If I have another one, I'm doing a home birth. I wish I had listened to you and done it at home. I could have just stayed home and done everything there."

That is the power of breaking down your fears. She embraced the pain, worked through her fears, and had her VBAC. It was a beautiful, empowering experience.

FAST, FURIOUS, AND GLORIOUS

This mom was 40 years old when she reached out to me. She had become pregnant unexpectedly by her partner, and although she had already given birth twice, both had been in hospitals. She didn't like the way her past birth experiences had gone—there had been elements of abuse, but she had still managed to have successful vaginal births each time. She had been following my content and listening to my podcast, and after watching my work, she knew she was going to do things differently this time around. She wanted a different kind of birth—one that would honor her body, experience, and choices.

She knew that if she chose a hospital again at 40 years old, she would be treated differently. However, she didn't want that because she was an extremely healthy 40-year-old woman, so together, we empowered her and educated her partner.

I remember joking, "Your first two were pretty quick hospital births, so if you stay home this time and avoid fear or intervention, I bet it'll happen really fast. It might just be you, your partner, and me."

I wasn't sure if she liked the idea at first, but she thought about it for a moment and said, "You know what? That would actually be a dream."

She loved the midwives I introduced her to, and everything seemed to be lining up beautifully for her birth. Then, one day, her husband called me around six in the morning. She had woken up to go to the bathroom, and while on the toilet, her water broke. The contractions came on strong and fast. I could hear her in the background, and her partner said, "It's pretty intense right now." I told him I'd be there in five minutes, though I lived about 14 minutes away.

In my rush, I grabbed my camera because I knew she didn't have any pictures or videos of her first two births and I wanted her to capture this experience. I grabbed my peanut ball and doula bag and ran out the door—without shoes, as I later realized!

When I got to her house, I set everything up as quickly as I could. Her two daughters, eight and six, were sitting on the stairs, looking worried, but their mom had asked them to stay outside of the room with their grandma because she was concerned they might get scared. I reassured them, saying, "She's so good. She's perfect. And your baby sister is perfect, too. Everything's going to be okay."

I set up the camera so the mama could capture the memory of this incredible birth. As I got everything ready, I quickly realized she was already pushing! Her body had taken over, and I knew the baby was coming soon. I called the midwife and put her on speakerphone. "You need to come now," I said, "She's having the baby."

Sure enough, just 57 minutes after the mother's first contraction, her baby was born. She fully surrendered to the process, and her body did exactly what it was meant to do. I encouraged her to reach down and grab her baby, but she was still in shock from the birth happening so fast. I placed the baby on her chest, and you could see the awe in her eyes. It had all happened so fast!

The midwife arrived shortly after, and the placenta was born. Then we went to get the mother's older daughters to introduce them to their new baby sister. It was such a beautiful, heart-warming moment. The girls came in and surrounded their mom on the bed, witnessing her power in the room where she had brought life into the world.

I find that family-centered births like these are powerful, especially for daughters. They get to witness their mother's strength and God-given ability to give birth, and that experience will give them confidence for when their time comes. It's a cycle of empowerment and belief in the body's capability that carries forward.

The birth was perfect and beautiful. As I looked at her, I couldn't help but think that if she had chosen a hospital, she likely wouldn't have made it in time—she might have had the baby in the car! This is why I love home births. You don't have to rush anywhere. You just stay home, and you have your baby, surrounded by peace and love.

That was fast, furious, and glorious.

ON GOD'S TIME

Timing your birth, timing your contractions—there's so much emphasis on time. Why? Why do we put a clock on a mother after her water breaks and pressure her body to labor or deliver within a specific timeframe? Yes, the risk of infection increases, but not significantly if there are no cervical checks or vaginal insertions.

This story is about a 45-year-old first-time mother who contacted me when she was ten weeks pregnant. She wanted to work through her fears and trust that her age would not dictate that she needed to birth in a hospital. I empowered her, educated her, and worked through her fears. In the end, however, she was still treated as high-risk simply because of her age and despite her incredibly healthy lifestyle. I wish it hadn't been that way, because her birth was beautiful.

Her midwives made her see a maternal-fetal medicine doctor, something I didn't find out until the end of her pregnancy. When she was 38 weeks along, she called me in tears. The doctors had told her that her fluid levels were too high, implying a risk of diabetes or other issues. However, her levels were actually within the normal range. I assured her that it could be something as simple as the baby having just peed before the scan—ultrasounds aren't 100% accurate, and that's why we must not put so much weight on them. That one ultrasound derailed her emotional preparation. She was told that if her fluid levels didn't drop by the next week, she'd have to be induced. That was a Wednesday, and by Friday, she would be 39 weeks.

I told her to wait until Monday for another scan. Something

in me felt that she might go into labor naturally before then and would still get her home birth. However, as you can imagine, the stress took a toll. She couldn't sleep or relax, and she became stuck in a heightened state of anxiety.

Around midnight on Friday, she called to say her water had broken. I told her to rest and that it's completely normal for contractions not to start for 12 to 24 hours, so she should sleep, hydrate, and prepare. The next morning, she told me she was starting to feel some sensations, so I came over. It was about 12 hours after her water had broken. She was experiencing early labor patterns, with contractions ranging from 20 minutes apart, to five, to ten, to 30—completely sporadic. I assured her that this didn't matter. She needed to sleep and conserve energy because she was exhausted.

We went for a walk in the beautiful weather, which sped things up a little, but she was still exhausted. I encouraged her to nap. Each time she fell asleep, the labor progressed more, becoming more intense. In the evening, her friend came over, and her husband rested in the living room while we stayed in the bedroom. She was laboring beautifully—on the toilet, shaking, growling, and surrendering to the process.

Then she asked me, "Why is it not working?"

"What do you mean?" I asked. "Your body's doing it."

"Why am I not pushing?" she said. "Why isn't it happening?"

She was in her head. That's what happens when we get too tired. Even in labor, sleep is your best weapon. The midwives started mentioning the 24-hour clock since her waters had been broken for that long.

"If she doesn't have the baby by noon tomorrow, we may have to transfer," they said.

I knew she could do it despite now being "observed" and having to perform while sleep-deprived. I suggested we blow up the birth pool and get her into the water. She labored in the pool, but the contractions slowed down, which made her worry. I reminded her that when contractions slow down, it often means her body is tired and her baby is resting. She needed to do the same. She couldn't rest, though, as she was too fixated on the clock the midwives had put her on. She didn't want to transfer to the hospital.

Eventually, she got out of the pool, still trying to surrender to the process. We tried every position imaginable—squatting, moving, anything to progress—but she was utterly exhausted.

Finally, she agreed to a cervical check. The midwife told her, "Your baby is right here. You're complete. You can push with the next contraction."

However, something inside the mother had shifted—a disconnect. "How long has my baby been there?" she wondered. "Am I damaging my baby? Why isn't my body pushing?"

Then her contractions stopped altogether. This happens sometimes when a mother gets too exhausted. It's called the rest phase—right before you push, your body and baby rest. This time, though, instead of resting, there was pressure to get things moving again with tinctures and pumping. In my heart, I knew she just needed sleep.

Your body labors the baby down, and then it pauses. There's nothing wrong with it. That rest is a natural part of the process— a moment for the baby to rest before traveling through the birth canal and a moment for the mother to gather strength for the final push. When you are fearful, you block the oxytocin flow. The mother had felt no fear up until that point.

Eventually, she pushed her baby out without any contractions —something rarely seen. However, pushing without contractions can damage your pelvic floor. That's why I always recommend not rushing the process and avoiding coached pushing.

If you're put on a clock to measure how long it's been since your water broke, remember that as long as you're not getting cervical checks and you don't have a fever, you can continue laboring naturally. Hydrate, trust the process, and let your baby come in God's time.

This mother got her home birth—pushing her baby out without the full strength of her uterus. It was beautiful to witness, but the trauma she experienced was due to being placed on a clock, preventing her from resting and relaxing.

Always ask your birth team how long they will let you labor if your membranes rupture. Rest is key. Trust your body. Your baby will come when the time is right—in God's time.

AN EMPOWERED REDEMPTION

This mama had her first home birth but experienced trauma when her baby got stuck—what practitioners call "shoulder dystocia." While many fear this situation, it doesn't need to be feared at all. It's just the absence of movement, and knowing how to manage it with maneuvers is key.

When she shared her birth story with me, she described how her baby got stuck while she was laboring in the pool. Her midwife made her get out, and when the baby finally emerged, he was lifeless and wasn't breathing. He had to be resuscitated, and the whole experience was very traumatic. Her parents were present, as well as her boyfriend, and everyone was panicking. Amidst all this, the oxytocin wasn't flowing as it should. Cortisol, the stress hormone, had likely taken over, causing her to tense up during pushing.

We broke down her first birth experience and worked through many of her fears. In examining the root of it all, we started with her early beliefs about birth. She told me about how her mother would always talk about tearing, how excruciating it was, and how she tore so much. However, her mother had given birth in a hospital, and I explained that hospital environments often contribute to such outcomes. I also addressed her fear of tearing directly.

She had been using primrose oil, inserting it vaginally, and taking it orally. Primrose oil tends to thin the membranes of the amniotic sac, which often leads to labor starting with the water breaking. If the water breaks before the baby is in the optimal position, the baby may end up in a less-than-ideal position for birth. This doesn't mean the baby is "stuck," but it does mean the baby might need more movement from the mother to get into a better position. I believe that's what happened during her first birth, given that she was using various natural induction methods. When the baby's head emerged, but the body didn't follow immediately, the midwife panicked, which caused the mother to panic as well. The tension built, and the midwife made her get out of the pool, which only added to the chaos.

The baby eventually came, but the birth needn't have gone that way.

For her second birth—her beautiful redemption—we discussed avoiding any kind of induction unless absolutely necessary. We agreed to let her body go beyond her due date if that was what was required. Then, one night around eleven o'clock, she messaged me, saying her water had broken. I told her to get some rest and let me know if she needed me. About an hour later, she said things were getting pretty intense, so I went to her.

When I arrived, she was sitting on the toilet, rocking back and forth but smiling. She was ready—so ready for her redemption—and I had reassured her it would be different this time. She was going to breathe her baby down and stay relaxed once the head emerged. The absence of contractions, which had caused tension in her last birth, wasn't going to affect this one.

This time, she would be bathed in oxytocin. She was going to surrender fully to her body, trusting that the next contraction would bring the force needed to push her little baby girl out. She continued rocking on the toilet, smiling as she embraced each wave. Finally, she said, "I think I want to get in the tub," and I helped her into the bath. There, she smiled even more, talking to her baby girl and roaring through each surge of labor when she needed to. It was incredibly powerful to witness.

As her baby began to emerge, she surrendered fully. The head came out, and her husband kissed her, telling her to stay calm and reassuring her that everything was perfect. With the next contraction and the power of her uterus, her baby girl was born and placed on her chest, where the infant let out a loud cry.

That moment healed so much trauma, not only for the mother but for her parents, who had been anxiously waiting in the guest room next door. They had heard it all, and I believe it healed their trauma as well.

It was a beautiful redemption—showing that if you can be empowered and educated the first time around, you don't need to go through the trauma. I want every mother to trust her body, to let herself be bathed in oxytocin, and to smile and laugh throughout the experience. This doesn't mean it will be pain free, but you can surrender completely to the process.

True redemption is possible.

A BORROWED HOUSE

I knew this woman from social media. She was so sweet, and we had been communicating back and forth for a few years but had never met in person. She let me know that she was coming to Austin for the birth of her third daughter. They had moved since her second daughter's birth, but they loved her Austin midwife so much that they just wanted to be back here to birth her baby. They had rented an Airbnb where the owners lived upstairs, but she and her husband didn't think this would be a problem since she intended to use a birth center.

She messaged me a week before her birth to let me know that "some bad stuff" had happened with the birth center, and the midwife no longer had access to it. I gave her my number so that I could help calm her down. Being 38 weeks pregnant and highly stressed was not conducive to a healthy birth.

When I spoke with her, I could hear the fear and panic in her voice. Something came over me, and I said, "I will just come help you when you go into labor. I live ten minutes from your Airbnb." I didn't know at the time that the owners lived upstairs.

The mother began having prodromal labor on and off for a few nights and was finding it hard to sleep from the stress and the uncomfortable bed in the rented space. I went to her to help her get a really deep nap by massaging her and leaving some tools with her. That's when I could tell she was resisting something. Her children were lovely; they wanted to help her and were ready to step up to that task, so I knew she wasn't holding back for them. That's when I found out: "The owners live upstairs," she told me right before I left her place at 4 a.m.

When I got home, I couldn't stop thinking about her not releasing. This was her element. She had birthed at home before. I could tell she was going to exhaust herself with this start-and-stop labor if she remained in that space. The following morning, when I checked on her, she was still having contractions eight to ten minutes apart (she wasn't timing them; she just could sense that this was about where they were).

I felt God nudge me with an urge to help her. She was not my client. She was just a friend on the internet. The power of God will move you if you listen, though. As my husband and I were sitting on our couch, I asked him, "Can a woman come to our house to have a baby?"

I could tell that he was studying my expression to see if I was serious. After thinking about it, he replied in the same tone he would have used if I had just asked him if our daughter could have a play date, "Sure, why not? We need to pick up the house, though. It's a mess." I love him. I didn't know how he would react, but I knew God had a hand in all of this, so, of course, my husband was on board.

I messaged her: "Come to my house… Here is the address… Let me know when the sensations pick up, and you feel you need the space to relax into them. I will set the guest room up like I did for my own home birth, and your daughters can sleep in Adeline's room." Normally, it would be insane to offer up your home to someone for a home birth, but I knew that was the only way this mother would actually be able to release and let go.

She texted me around 7 p.m. that they were heading to get dinner and the sensations were picking up quite a bit, so they would most likely be at my house shortly after dinner. I had set the space for her and let the midwife know my address. The midwife was at another birth 45 minutes away, so she told me that she would send someone closer to my house until she could get there.

As soon as Mom and Dad arrived and got the kids to bed in Adeline's room, you could see the release on her face. They put on their favorite music and were laughing and joking. She would pause to have a surge and then would go right back to having fun and playing music with her husband. I knew they were BOTH exhausted, so I suggested that she lie in the bed (my guest bed is heavenly!) to get some rest. She lay down with her husband, and I gave her a peanut ball to rest with. They were instantly excited about how much more comfortable the bed was.

They napped for a good hour, and then the surges began to intensify. She would get up and rock and sway to them. Her husband was her doula; I got to just document the birth for them, something she hadn't been able to do with her other births. My husband was in our master bedroom with our sleeping toddler and baby, so this was my first time not having to worry about being away from my babies while at a birth.

Finally, the rest of the midwife team arrived, and Mama danced and swayed through each surge, talking to herself, praising God, and telling herself out loud, "You can do this. You can do this."

Her two-year-old and my one-year-old had woken up and were playing with each other in my living room, so I took on the role of entertaining them while Mama labored. As she got closer to transition, the noises intensified, and my four-year-old wanted to see what was happening. She pulled her little chair into the hallway and watched with awe. The midwife held the mother's two-year-old on her lap. She had been the midwife for her birth as well. It was the most beautiful thing to witness. Everyone was just holding space for this mother while she stood and held onto her husband.

Her surges became pushy. As she birthed her beautiful baby girl next to the bed, Adeline stood and began singing "Amazing Grace." That is the power of witnessing birth: a four-year-old was so overcome with emotion that she had to sing. I wept.

Of course, the mother and father were exhausted, so I took care of them postpartum, and then they returned to their Airbnb with their precious bundle. I will never forget the feeling I had of "just have her come have the baby here." It changed a lot of lives that day. This is a testament to how much influence the environment has on your birth. Get somewhere you feel safe, where you can release.

CONCLUSION

As we come to the end of this journey, I hope you have gained a new perspective on birth—one rooted in faith, knowledge, and empowerment. Undisturbed physiological birth isn't just a possibility; it's how our bodies were designed to work. Through the ups and downs of pregnancy and labor, trusting God and His creation is key to experiencing the fullness of birth as it was meant to be.

Whether you're preparing for your first birth, seeking healing after a difficult experience, or supporting others as they bring life into the world as a doula or midwife, remember that birth is not something to be feared or managed. It is a divine gift. With the right preparation, a strong support system, and unwavering faith, you can embrace your birth with confidence, knowing that your body and your baby are capable of incredible things. My prayer is that you move forward from here empowered, equipped, and ready to embrace the miracle of birth as God intended.

CONCLUSION

If you wish to book one-on-one coaching with me
or use any of my other services, visit my website,
www.EmmyRobbinDoula.com. If you want to hear more
in-depth birth stories and fun discussions, you can listen
to my podcast, *Empowered Birth Love and Life*.

THANK YOU FOR READING MY BOOK!

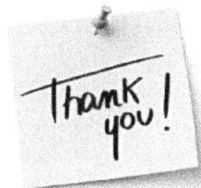

Thank you so much for buying my book!
Scan the QR code to get a 100% off coupon
to one of my masterminds!

Scan the QR Code:

SCAN ME

I appreciate your interest in my book, and value your feedback
as it helps me improve future versions.
I would appreciate it if you could leave your invaluable review
on Amazon.com with your feedback.
Thank you!

www.ingramcontent.com/pod-product-compliance
Lightning Source LLC
Chambersburg PA
CBHW031437270326
41930CB00007B/744